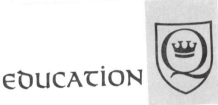

NUTRITION
AND
DISEASE
LOOKING
FOR THE
LINK
D.J. ARNESON

FRANKLIN WATTS
NEW YORK/ CHICAGO/ LONDON/ TORONTO/ SYDNEY
A VENTURE BOOK

Photographs copyright ©: The Bettmann Archive: pp. 4, 8; Photo
Researchers, Inc.: pp. 9 (Omikron), 41 top (SPL), 41 bottom (Thomas
England), 55 (Bettye Lane), 114 (Myron Wood); UPI/Bettmann
Newsphotos: p. 117; AP/Wide World Photos: pp. 30, 118; Gamma-Liaison:
p. 52; Rothco Cartoons: pp. 112 top (Boileau), 112 bottom (Wicks).
Diagram copyright © Vantage Art

Library of Congress Cataloging-in-Publication Data

Arneson, D. J.
    Nutrition and disease / by D.J. Arneson.
        p.   cm.— (A Venture book)
    Includes bibliographical references (p.   ) and index.
    Summary: Discusses the functions of the body's systems, including
skeletal, muscular, and nervous; and examines the relationship
between nutrition and breakdowns in body systems and diseases.
    ISBN 0-531-12504-1
    1. Nutrition—Juvenile literature. 2. Nutritionally induced
diseases—Juvenile literature. [1. Nutrition. 2. Nutritionally
induced diseases.]   I. Title.
QP141.A68   1992
612.3—dc20   92-14473 CIP AC

CONTENTS

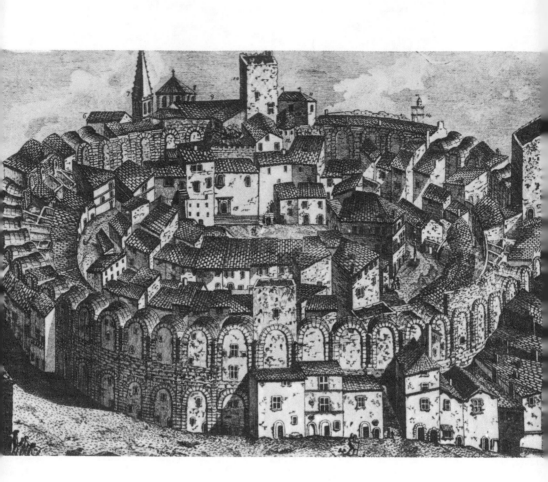

*European towns in the Middle Ages were so
heavily fortified that during times of war
it was difficult to get food and water brought in
from outside sources. This often resulted
in a scarcity of food for the inhabitants.*

INTRODUCTION

People lived in nutritional harmony with nature from the time they first gathered food in the wild to the development of agriculture, which had its beginnings about 10,000 years ago. The transition from the need to find food and the ability to grow food took hundreds of thousands of years.[1] It was so gradual that by the time crop cultivation and the domestication of animals replaced hunting and gathering, available foods continued to meet the nutritional needs of the human diet. What people did not grow or raise themselves was available through trade. Instances of nutrition-related disease were too far apart and on too small a scale for people to make any connection between the disease and food.

In Europe in the Middle Ages, many people lived in towns and cities. They had to depend on food brought in from the countryside. In times of war, these population centers were often surrounded by their enemies in sieges—blockades designed to defeat the encircled city by cutting off supplies of food and water. During long sieges many people in the encircled cities found themselves growing weaker. Their health slowly deteriorated. They began to suffer from fatigue, body aches, pain when making simple movements, swollen cheeks, rotting gums, falling teeth, and splotchy purple bruises on their skin. Many died, but the cause of death was not always simple starvation. Some deaths were the consequence of scurvy, a disease that resulted from a lack of certain kinds of food—mainly fresh produce—in the diet. Nobody made the connection at the time between the scarcity of fruits and vegetables and the epidemic illness and death because it was not known that certain foods or constituents of foods were essential to health and life. Scurvy and its causes were unknown.

During the age of exploration, new discoveries in the art of seafaring made it possible for ships to venture farther from land than ever before. The sailors of the 1500s spent long periods at sea. Like the citizens of the beseiged cities, the ships' crews began to suffer common symptoms of fatigue, pain, rotting gums, and more. They too were unaware that the illness was associated with their diet.

Later, as voyages stretched over months and even years, the British Royal Navy concocted a diet for its sailors that would not spoil when carried for long periods. Each man received a standard daily ration of 4,000 calories. This included a pound of hard biscuits; about a pound of salt meat or dried fish; a few ounces of butter, cheese, or dried peas; and a gallon of beer to drink. It was believed that this diet would keep a sailor in good health. The tragic discovery was that it led to illness and death. Sailors' gums bled easily and rotted, their skin became covered with purple blotches, and their teeth fell out as they stumbled about on cold, hard, swollen legs. In about twenty years, as many as 10,000 sailors of the Royal Navy died of scurvy, a disease we now know is caused by a deficiency of ascorbic acid—vitamin C—in the diet.[2]

Scurvy wasn't limited to British sailors. Vasco da Gama, the Portuguese explorer, lost 100 out of 160 of his crew on a voyage, and other long-distance navigators' crews fared as poorly.

In the late 1700s, James Lind, a Scottish surgeon, tried giving lime juice—an excellent source of vitamin C, although he didn't know it—to sailors who had developed scurvy. The results were good, and scurvy began to disappear. Since that time, British sailors have been known as "limeys," although Lind may have actually used lemon or orange juice.

Scurvy wasn't the only seafaring, nutrition-related disease of the era, and Western sailors weren't the only victims. Japan's powerful navy also sailed out to sea for long periods. A major component of a Japanese sailor's diet was polished rice, rice with its natural hull removed. Long-distance sailors often suffered from stiffness, paralysis, and pain and slowly wasted away. Sometimes as many as two-thirds of a crew died. Something was missing in the men's diets. What wasn't known was that vitamins contained in the hull—particularly vitamin B_1 (thiamine)—are removed when rice is polished. Just as a deficiency of vitamin C caused scurvy, the lack of vitamin B_1 in the diet caused this disease, beriberi. The disease was controlled when the sailors' diet was changed to include the nutrients removed when the rice was polished.

During the Depression in the United States many years later, thousands of people in the South died of pellagra. Also known as the "4 Ds" for its associated conditions of diarrhea, dermatitis, dementia, and, finally, death, pellagra was caused by a deficiency of niacin (vitamin B_3) in the typical diet of corn products such as cornbread, hominy, and grits. Corn is low in niacin. Preventive measures that included niacin-rich foods such as liver, eggs, milk, and meat in the diet eliminated the problem.

Rickets, a disease primarily of infants and children that leads to abnormal bone formation, is caused

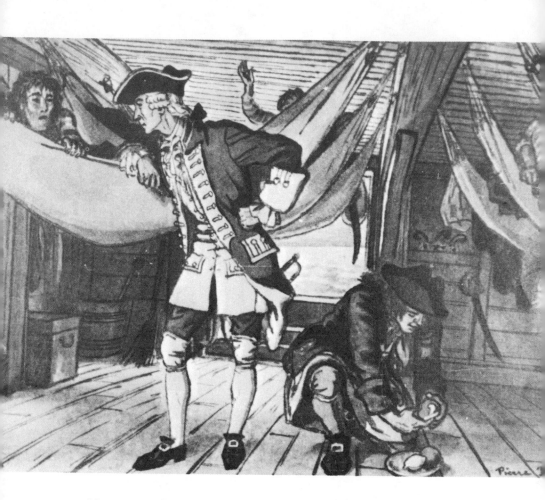

Above: *Sir James Lind (1716–1794), "the father of naval hygiene in England," experimented with remedies for scurvy. These experiments resulted in the British naval order to supply sailors with lemon juice.*

Right: *This Sumatran child's bow-legged condition is due to a deficiency of vitamin D in her diet.*

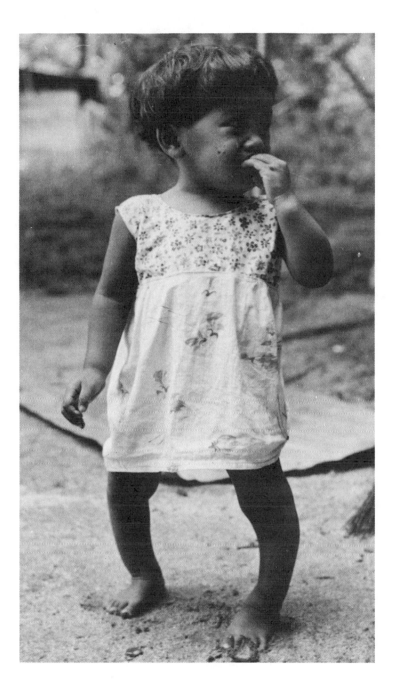

by a deficiency of vitamin D. Vitamin D, which is essential for the absorption of calcium for bone growth, is produced naturally in the skin when exposed to sunlight. Rickets was prevalent in the United States in the early part of the twentieth century, particularly in northern states where children were bundled up for much of the year. The addition of vitamin D to milk eliminated the problem.

Also in this century, a part of the American Midwest was known as the "goiter belt" because of a high rate of goiter, a thyroid gland condition that resulted from a deficiency of iodine in the diet. The usual sources of iodine, particularly seafood, were unavailable in the region. Federal legislation requiring that iodine be added to salt, a food seasoning used by most people, virtually eliminated the problem.

Episodes like these led to the recognition of a connection between nutrition and disease, but it took many years before controlled scientific experiments began to unravel the mysteries of nutrition.

Research has proved there are substantial links between nutrition and health. Much has been learned, but the significance and extent of the connections are not yet fully known. The information we have is sometimes compromised by conflicting interpretations of data. Faced with a lack of complete, undisputed evidence, conflicting interpretations of information, contradictory claims, and much personal opinion, many people are puzzled about nutrition–disease connections.

Becoming familiar with the pieces of a puzzle is the first step to making intelligent decisions regarding the whole. In trying to understand the link between nutrition and disease, we start with how the body works and what role nutrition plays in keeping the body working correctly.

PART I
THE BODY

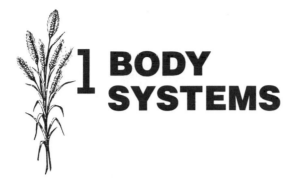

1 BODY SYSTEMS

Your body is a collection of many organs and systems working together. You hear, see, think, move, breathe, grow, digest, sweat, remember, heal, fight infection, store energy, get rid of wastes, and much more. Everything works smoothly, in unison, and with little or no conscious effort on your part.

Organs are specialized, individual parts. The brain, heart, lungs, and liver are organs. When several organs are linked together to perform a specific or organized task, they form a "system." The stomach, intestine, liver, and some other organs make up the digestive system, for example. The human body is all the organs and systems taken together. For the body to survive, all of its systems must work together. Most systems work automatically—you don't have to tell them what to do, and you couldn't even if you tried. Other systems are under your control—you can start or stop what they do at will.

SKELETAL SYSTEM

The skeleton, the body's frame, is made up of 206 connected bones that act like the steel girders that support a tall building. Without its frame, the building would collapse; without a skeleton, you could not sit, stand up, or even move.

Your skeleton supports you, gives your body its basic shape, protects vital organs like your brain, heart, and lungs from injury, and holds your muscles in place so they can move your whole body or its parts.

The femur or thigh bone is the largest bone in the body. Long, thick, heavy, and very strong, it requires the body's largest muscles to move it. The body's smallest bones are three tiny structures in the inner ear so delicate that a puff of wind against the eardrum can move them.

Bones are made up largely of calcium. Ninety percent of the body's calcium is stored in the skeleton. Bone is hard and dense. Long bones like the bones of your legs, arms, toes, and fingers are hollow and filled with marrow, a spongy specialized tissue that makes red and white blood cells. Other types of bone are short bones—the wrist bones and kneecaps, for example; flat bones—the ribs, skull, sternum, hips, and shoulder blades; and irregular bones—the bones of the face and vertebrae.

Bones are held together in joints by elastic tissue called ligaments. The ligaments permit slight movement in the joints of some bones like the ribs, or full, hinged movement as with the knees or elbows. Bone ends are protected from shock by a covering of cartilage, a soft tissue.

MUSCULAR SYSTEM

Over 600 muscles, the body's "motors," make up 35 to 40 percent of the body's weight. They move bones and organs by contracting and relaxing. Each muscle is separate, although most muscles work in groups.

Muscle tissue consists of rows of threadlike cells or fibers held together in protective sheaths. The fibers contract when stimulated, shortening muscle tissue. If the muscle is connected to a bone, the bone moves. If the muscle surrounds a space, as it does in the heart and intestines, the space is squeezed smaller and anything inside the space is forced to move. Swallowing is an example. As the throat muscles contract, food or saliva is forced down into the esophagus. Muscle energy comes from nutrients carried in the bloodstream.

There are three types of muscle tissue—skeletal muscle, smooth muscle, and cardiac muscle. Skeletal muscle moves bones and certain organs, like the eyes and tongue. It encloses and protects the abdominal organs. It is attached to bones by tendon, a strong, elastic tissue. Most skeletal muscles are arranged in opposing pairs so that when one contracts, the other relaxes. Skeletal muscle movement is voluntary.

Voluntary muscles are under your control. Turning your head, moving your fingers, and running are voluntary movements. Some voluntary muscle movements like preventing yourself from falling by regaining your balance are reflexes and are controlled by the nervous system.

Smooth muscle movement is involuntary and is controlled by automatic mechanisms operating in the brain. The smooth muscles of the heart, blood vessels, and intestines work automatically.

Cardiac muscle is a specialized smooth muscle found only in the heart.

NERVOUS SYSTEM

All body systems must be connected and coordinated to function in unison. The nervous system is the control and communication network that keeps all the other systems working together. It also brings in information from the world around you.

The nervous system consists of the central nervous system—the brain and spinal cord; the peripheral nervous system—cranial (skull) and spinal nerves; and the autonomic nervous system—specialized peripheral nerves. Voluntary actions are controlled through the central nervous system. Involuntary actions, such as heartbeat and breathing, are controlled by the autonomic nervous system. Both may utilize the nerves of the peripheral nervous system.

The brain is the master control center. Its many areas work simultaneously at thousands of different tasks. Specific areas control everything the body does. Thinking is done in the front part of the cerebrum, the largest, uppermost part of the brain. Temporal lobes above the ears interpret sound, and vision is interpreted at the back of the cerebrum.

Nerve fibers made up of specialized cells carry "messages" in the form of electrical impulses between the brain and every part of the body. Specialized nerve cells in the eyes, ears, skin, nose, and other sensitive organs convert light, sound, heat or cold, pressure, and smell into signals for the brain to interpret and then choose reactions.

CIRCULATORY SYSTEM

The circulatory system consists of the heart and a closed network of blood vessels to transport blood to all parts of the body. End to end, the system of blood vessels would circle the globe more than twice.

Blood vessels are grouped by function. Arteries carry blood from the heart to all parts of the body. Capillaries—microscopically small tubes with walls a single cell thick—carry blood from tiny arteries (arterioles) to body cells and return it to tiny veins (venules). Veins carry blood from the body back to the heart.

Blood is made of plasma, a liquid that is 90 percent water, and specialized cells called corpuscles. Red corpuscles, which transport oxygen, turn arterial blood bright red because they are rich in iron and oxygen. Venous blood is depleted of oxygen and has a bluish color. White corpuscles fight infection by destroying pathogens, or disease-causing organisms. There are several types of corpuscles, and these are a large part of the immune system. Cell fragments called platelets prevent bleeding by causing blood to clot.

Blood stays in the capillaries, but the nutrients, hormones, and oxygen it carries pass through the thin capillary walls into a slightly salty fluid that surrounds all living body cells. The body cells absorb the materials they need from the solution and transfer wastes back into it. The wastes pass through the capillary walls into the bloodstream and are carried to the liver, lungs, kidneys, skin, and intestines for excretion.

The heart is a four-chambered muscular pump, slightly larger than a fist, that forces blood through the circulatory system. It is located between the lungs, just to the left of the breastbone. It beats an average of 72 times a minute and circulates about 650,000 gallons of blood in one year.

The heart is really two pumps, separated by a partition through the center of the organ. Each side has two chambers, an atrium on top and a ventricle below. Each side beats separately with a brief rest between beats.

The right atrium receives venous blood returning from the body. It contracts to send the blood into the right ventricle, which pumps it to the lungs for oxygenation. Oxygenated blood already in the lung's capillaries is forced back into the left atrium of the heart. It then goes to the left ventricle, which pumps it through arteries to the body.

Onc-way valves in each heart chamber prevent blood from flowing backward. When a chamber contracts, its entrance valve closes and its exit valve opens.

The heartbeat is controlled by the autonomic nervous system, which monitors the body's needs for oxygen. A demand for more oxygen speeds up the heart; resting slows it down. The heart has its own blood supply. When that blood supply is interrupted, the heart suffers a myocardial infarction, or "heart attack."

RESPIRATORY SYSTEM

The function of the respiratory system is to oxygenate blood and remove carbon dioxide and water to be expelled in the breath.

Air enters and leaves the respiratory system when you breathe. Inhalation draws oxygen-rich air into the nose, through the nasal cavities, down the windpipe (trachea), and into the lungs located inside the chest cavity. Branchlike air tubes called bronchi carry the air to tiny alveoli (air sacs), where blood-filled capillaries exchange oxygen and carbon dioxide. Waste-laden air is exhaled back into the atmosphere. The inhalation-exhalation cycle is repeated an average of twenty times a minute.

Air is pumped by the action of the diaphragm, a dome-shaped sheet of muscle that separates the chest and abdominal cavities. On inhalation the diaphragm contracts downward and the chest walls expand to increase the size of the chest cavity, reducing the air pressure inside the lungs. Atmospheric air under greater pressure rushes into the lungs. When the diaphragm relaxes, the dome rises, the chest compresses, inside air pressure increases, and the air rushes out.

Normal breathing is controlled automatically by the brain, but the depth and rate of breathing can be voluntarily controlled for short periods, as in long-distance running or meditation.

DIGESTIVE SYSTEM

All activity requires energy. The body produces energy by oxidizing (chemically burning) sugars and fats from digested food in its cells.

The digestive system (the alimentary canal) is made up of the mouth, esophagus, stomach, small and large intestines, and the accessory organs of digestion, which are the liver, gallbladder, and pancreas.

Food is chewed and mixed with a digestive juice (saliva) and enzymes in the mouth. Swallowing forces the softened food down the esophagus and into the stomach. Stronger digestive juices and enzymes are added as the stomach churns it into liquid. The liquid enters the small intestine, where more digestive juices are added, breaking it down into simpler forms for use.

The small intestine is lined with a velvety-looking covering of fingerlike projections called villi. Nutrients and water in the intestine are absorbed into the bloodstream through villi walls and are then transported to the cells of the body for use or storage.

Most nutrients have been absorbed by the time material in the digestive tract reaches the large intestine. The remaining material plus other waste products are held in the lower part of the large intestine for elimination.

The liver, an accessory organ of digestion, is one of the body's most complex organs. It is located beneath the diaphragm, next to the stomach. About one and a half quarts of blood enter the liver every minute through its double blood supply. One blood supply brings oxygen-rich blood from the lungs, and the other brings nutrients and raw materials from the digestive tract.

19

The liver is a true chemical factory. Its major functions are to store glucose, manufacture blood products, treat wastes, change fats so they can be used, make bile to break down fats, remove toxic substances from the blood, and make the material that prevents blood from clotting.

The gallbladder, a small, muscular sac behind the liver, receives the bile and stores it for release as needed.

The pancreas, a gland behind the stomach, secretes a strong digestive juice that aids in the breakdown of food in the stomach. It is also responsible for the production of insulin, which controls the amount of sugar in the blood.

REPRODUCTIVE SYSTEM

Humans reproduce through specialized male and female cells. The male cells—spermatozoa, or sperm—are produced in glands called testes. The female cells—ova, or eggs—are formed in glands called ovaries.

An egg takes about one month to mature. Alternating ovaries produce one egg approximately every twenty-eight days—the length of the female menstrual cycle. The egg leaves the ovary and travels through a fallopian tube to enter the top of the uterus, a muscular organ in the lower part of a woman's abdomen. The walls of the uterus have a rich supply of blood vessels. Fertilization takes place in the uterus when a single sperm penetrates the wall of a mature egg. Chromosomes carrying genetic instructions from each parent are combined and a single cell called a zygote is formed. The zygote immediately begins a process of division and attaches to the uterine wall, where it is nourished by nutrients from the mother's blood supply. Physical characteristics such as size, shape, skin, and eye and hair color are a few of the many thousands of bits of information carried in reproductive cells. The individual formed from the union will display some characteristics of each parent. In about three months the growing offspring, or fetus, resembles an infant. In about nine months the fetus is fully developed and ready to be born.

GLANDULAR SYSTEM

Glands are organs that produce specialized chemical substances the body uses to perform certain functions. External secretions such as digestive juices, tears, and sweat do their work directly. Internal secretions (hormones) are carried in the bloodstream to other parts of the body where they act as chemical messengers by instructing an organ to work. Hormones often work jointly with the nervous system to regulate and control body activities.

The pituitary gland, located deep inside the brain, is called the "master gland" because its hormones stimulate other glands. Pituitary hormones regulate growth, reproductive organ development, smooth muscle activity, and other important functions.

The thyroid gland, located in the throat just below the "Adam's apple," produces hormones that affect growth, heart rate, body temperature, and other functions. The parathyroids, near the thyroid, regulate bone growth, muscles, and nerves.

Two adrenal glands (one on top of each kidney) secrete a variety of hormones affecting numerous body functions, from reproduction to breathing rate.

The pancreas lies behind the stomach and produces digestive juices and insulin, a hormone that controls blood sugar levels. It plays a role in the digestive system also.

Female ovaries and male testes produce hormones that affect appearance and the reproductive process.

21

The thymus is located in the upper chest. Its hormones help to stimulate the body's defenses against infection. The function of the pineal gland, a cone-shaped structure about one-fourth of an inch long deep inside the brain, is not fully known. Both these glands have roles in aging that are not completely understood.

URINARY SYSTEM

Burning nutrients for energy, for building tissue, and other activities creates wastes that must be eliminated. Many body systems get rid of wastes. The digestive system eliminates solid wastes and water (feces) from the large intestine. The respiratory system eliminates carbon dioxide and water in the breath. The skin eliminates water and some waste salts in sweat. The urinary system's function is to remove the waste products of metabolism from the liver and the blood. The urinary system then eliminates them from the body in the urine.

Two bean-shaped kidneys, one on each side of the body in the middle of the back under the diaphragm, are the urinary system's major organs. They act as filters to remove waste material from the blood. Each kidney is connected by a tube (ureter) to the urinary bladder. The bladder is a sac for collecting urine from the kidneys. When the bladder is full, nerves stimulate the urge to empty it by urinating. Urine passes from the bladder to the outside through another tube, the urethra.

The kidneys also help regulate the amount of water in the body.

SKIN (INTEGUMENTARY SYSTEM)

The skin—a continuous, flexible, protective barrier over the outside of the body—is the body's largest organ. Its many functions include preventing underlying tissues from drying out, keeping out bacteria and harmful substances, regulating body temperature, gathering information about the environment, eliminating certain wastes, and making vitamin D from sunlight.

Skin thickness varies with the kind of protection needed. The soles of the hands and feet are thick, for example, while eyelids are thin. Hair, nails, and sweat and oil glands seen at the surface originate in deeper layers of the skin.

The surface of the skin's firm outer layer, the epidermis, is made of flat, dead cells. They are formed from living cells that are pushed to the top by new cells that grow deeper in the epidermis. As dead, outer cells wear off, they are replaced by others.

The deepest layer of the epidermis contains cells that produce melanin, the pigment that gives skin color. Freckles are tiny patches of melanin.

Beneath the epidermis is the dermis, or "true skin." It contains elastic connective tissue, blood vessels, and nerves. The dermis lies on top of the subcutaneous (under the skin) layer. Sweat and oil glands and hair and nails originate in the dermis and subcutaneous layer. The subcutaneous layer contains fat that acts as insulation and can be burned by the body for energy.

Sweat glands pass perspiration (water and mineral wastes) onto the skin through tiny pores. As the water evaporates, it cools the body. Sebrum, an oily substance from oil glands, keeps hair soft.

SENSORY SYSTEMS

You see, hear, smell, and feel the world around you and even keep your balance by using sensory information that reaches you through your eyes, ears, nose, skin, and other sensory organs or receptors (specialized nerves).

23

Vision

The eye receives light reflected off objects you see. The light passes through a lens in the pupil and is focused on the retina at the back of the eyeball where nerve endings sense it and convert the sensations into electrical signals. The signals travel over the optic nerve to the brain, which translates the signals into images.

Hearing

Sound waves beating against your eardrums are converted to motion that travels over the tiny bones of the middle ear to the fluid-filled semicircular canals and cochlea of the inner ear. Nerves in the canals and cochlea sense movement in the fluid. Movement in the semicircular canals sends signals to the brain that are interpreted for equilibrium. Signals from sensors in the cochlea are translated by the brain as sound.

Smell and taste

Extremely tiny particles of material enter your nose when you breathe. When they touch specialized nerves inside the nose, chemical reactions produce signals that travel through a nerve to the brain. The brain interprets the signals as smells.

Chemicals in food stimulate areas of the tongue containing taste buds. Taste buds send signals to the brain which are interpreted as sweet, sour, salty, or bitter. Other familiar tastes are really associated with the sense of smell.

Feeling

Nerve endings in the skin and other parts of the body are sensitive to heat, cold, pressure, or pain. When stimulated, they send signals to the brain that are translated according to the stimulus. For example, an ice cube sends a signal of "cold," and a scratch sends a signal of "pain."

IMMUNITY

Immunity is a process rather than a system, although it is sometimes called the "immune system."[1] It is an individual's power to resist or overcome the effects of specific diseases or harmful agents that produce toxins, or poisons. The process is selective rather than general. That is, a person can be immune to one or many diseases, but immunity to one does not necessarily give immunity to another. A child can be immune to chicken pox and still be susceptible to measles.

Immunity is produced by chemical processes in the body that fight off the effects of pathogens (disease-producing microorganisms) before they begin. Pathogens contain substances that the body sees as antigens. When bacteria enter the body, the antigens they carry cause the body to produce antibodies. The antibodies destroy the invading bacteria or act on them so that white blood cells can destroy them. There are many different kinds of antigens, and each kind stimulates the body to produce an antibody that responds only to it.

There are two basic types of immunity—inherited immunity and acquired immunity. Inherited immunity is genetic. That humans don't get hog cholera is an example of inherited immunity. Acquired immunity can be natural or artificial. When antibodies in a mother's blood are transferred to her fetus, the developing fetus gains naturally acquired immunity. Naturally acquired immunity may also be gained as a result of having a disease. Once you have chicken pox, you won't have it again. When a person is vaccinated against a disease, he or she gains artificially acquired immunity.

When the immune system is deficient, the body cannot adequately defend itself against antigens. If the deficiency is severe, infection goes unchecked and serious illness or death may result.

AIDS (acquired immune deficiency syndrome) is a dramatic example of immune system deficiency. The invading virus (HIV, or human immunodeficiency virus) alters the body's ability to defend itself. Unprotected, the body is unable to fight off infections and eventually is overwhelmed and dies.

This complex collection of systems, parts, and functions comprise the human body. It is a machine, but one with an extraordinary difference—it is alive. Every cell and system of the human body is physically and physiologically united into a single, self-contained, self-aware, living organism biochemically energized by a process called nutrition. Whether the body lives in health or disease—or fails to survive at all—depends on the interrelationships among its organs and systems and on its underlying nutrition.

PART II
NUTRITION

The human body is a living organism. To survive, it must take in certain materials from the outside and change them into usable forms to get energy, grow, adapt, and reproduce. The materials, or nutrients, come from food. Nutrition is the movement of food and its usable forms into the body to keep it healthy.

The body and its many organs are capable of thousands of separate functions. The heart pumps blood, nerves sense the outside world, muscles extend and contract, lungs transfer oxygen and carbon dioxide, the stomach digests food, and the brain—like a central control system—plays a part in all of this. When everything is taken together, the whole body functions as if it were a single thing. In reality it is a collection of distinct organs and parts. When one part of the organism gets sick, the whole organism is affected, even though the person may be unaware of it until the sickness or disease is severe.

Certain nutrients are essential to life; the body will die without them. But the lack of an essential nutrient does not kill the body all at once the way a fast-acting poison would. When the body is denied a nutrient it needs to survive, it gets sick, beginning with the part that requires the missing nutrient. At

27

first the sickness may not be noticeable. Other body systems may compensate for the affected system, or the sick organ or system may continue to function, but at less than full speed. The body may live in a diseased state for many years. Think of a light bulb that gets only enough electricity to glow, but not enough to shine brightly the way it could if it were receiving all the energy it needed.

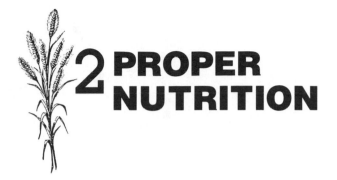

2 PROPER NUTRITION

The body is properly nourished when it gets the nutrients it needs in the right amounts to survive in good health; it is poorly nourished when it doesn't get what it needs. The difference between proper nutrition and poor nutrition is determined by what is in the foods we eat and whether it reaches the organs and systems that need it.

Each person has his or her own nutritional needs. Individual differences in the size, shape, and efficiency of digestive organs; in eating habits (frequency, amounts eaten, time taken to eat); and in amounts of various nutrients required determine what is right for that person.

The amount of food consumed is determined by the appetite, which is determined by what is available and by the appestat—a neural control center in the brain.[1] Psychological factors may also influence the appetite.

Eating patterns affect human nutrition, too. The common practice of skipping breakfast, for example, not only denies a person the direct nutritional benefits of the meal, but also causes fluctuations of blood sugar and insulin levels and increases percentages of fat and cholesterol in the body. A good breakfast also aids concentration and provides better appetite control.

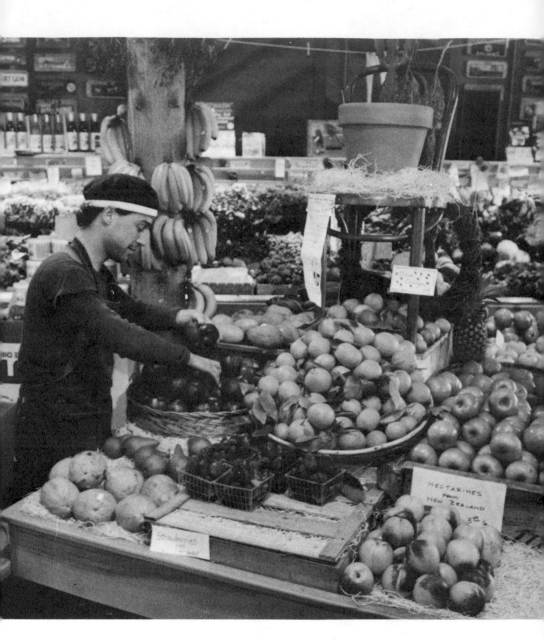

The variety of foods in this large supermarket
makes proper nutrition easy to achieve.

The various nutrients contained in food are all important; no single one by itself can support life and guarantee good health. Evidence suggests that some antinutrients—components of food that prevent the absorption of minerals and proteins into the body— are beneficial. They have been shown to retard the rise of blood sugar levels and may lessen the symptoms of a type of diabetes by increasing insulin receptor sensitivity. They also help to prevent heart disease by regulating cholesterol levels in the blood.

Nutrients enter the body in food. The vitamin C in the lime juice ingested by a British sailor, for example, does not float around as little specks in the juice, and the vitamin D added to milk is not visible. These vitamins—and all nutrients—are complex chemical forms locked together in the food. They must be broken down into simpler forms the body can use. Once broken down, they are transported throughout the body to where they are needed. They then undergo more change to produce heat, grow and repair tissue, resist infection, or perform whatever other function is needed for survival.

The processes that convert food are digestion, absorption, circulation, and metabolism—a chain of physical and chemical events. Physical changes in food are produced by grinding and churning caused by muscular movement. Chemical changes occur when digestive juices, or enzymes (substances that cause a chemical change without being changed themselves), are mixed with the food to break it down into other chemical forms. These changes take place within the digestive tract.

DIGESTION

Digestion is the conversion of food into substances the body can absorb and use. The process begins in the

31

mouth when a bite of food is ground into pulp by chewing. Salivary glands in the mouth secrete a watery substance, saliva, the first digestive juice to act on food. Saliva contains an enzyme, ptyalin, that breaks down carbohydrate, a nutrient. It also moistens the chewed food into a wet paste. Well-chewed food mixes better with saliva and is easier to swallow. Improper chewing lets large pieces of solid food pass into the stomach where it is harder to digest than smaller pieces.

Chewed food is forced to the back of the mouth, the pharynx, by the movement of the mouth and tongue. The mixture is moved from the pharynx into the esophagus and then to the stomach by peristalsis, an automatic, wavelike contraction and relaxation of the muscles of the digestive tract, also called the alimentary canal. Imagine the alimentary canal as a rubber tube partially filled with mud. Closing your hand around the top of the tube and squeezing forces the mud to slide down. Squeezing with your other hand below the first fist continues to push the mud down. Peristalsis is similar to this action, but is involuntary.

The stomach is a gourd-shaped ballooning of the digestive tract. Its principal functions are to store and churn food. Muscle valves, or sphincters, at each end open and close to allow food in and out. The stomach can hold up to a half-gallon of food and liquid.

The stomach's muscular walls churn the food while glands in the walls produce digestive juices, gastric juices, that mix with it. Gastric juices—mainly water, hydrochloric acid, and enzymes—further break down the food until it is reduced to a semi-liquid, or chyme. Depending on how much and what kind of food was eaten, the mixture remains in the stomach for one to four hours. Most liquids leave the stomach almost as soon as they enter. Very little actual digestion takes place in the stomach.

The churned liquid is released into the small intestine through the valve at the lower end of the stomach. Two accessory organs of digestion, the pancreas and the liver, are connected to the upper portion of the small intestine by small ducts. These accessory organs produce additional juices that aid in the process of digestion. The pancreas secretes pancreatic juice and the liver secretes bile. Bile is stored in the gallbladder before being released into the small intestine. Bile breaks down fat into small drops that are then broken down further by pancreatic juice.

The major work of digestion takes place in the upper end of the small intestine. Here the nutrients in food—carbohydrates, proteins, and fats—are broken down into simpler molecules (fundamental chemical compounds) so that they can be absorbed into the body. Carbohydrates are converted to sugar (glucose), proteins are converted to amino acids, and fats are converted to fatty acids and glycerol. Up to this point, food is still "outside" the body because the alimentary canal is actually a hollow tube running through the body. Once the chemically simplified nutrients pass through the walls of the small intestine, they are then truly inside the body. This process is absorption.

ABSORPTION

The small intestine is about twenty feet (6 m) long. Most of it is devoted to absorbing nutrients which now are in the form of molecules.

The walls of the small intestine are lined with millions of microscopically small villi—fingerlike projections. Their covering is only one cell layer thick. Cell walls are remarkably thin, semipermeable membranes. Certain food molecules can pass through them while others are helped through by special proteins in the cell membranes.

Inside the villi tiny veins and arteries are connected by capillaries, miniature tubes with walls that are also one cell thick. Food molecules that have passed through villi lining the small intestine are now absorbed into the bloodstream through the thin walls of the capillaries.

Most absorption of basic food material, water, and mineral salts takes place in the small intestine. Once in the bloodstream, these nutrients are transported throughout the body by the circulation of blood.

CIRCULATION

The body's circulatory system—the vast network of small to microscopically small tubes—circulates blood to all the body's living tissues, transporting raw materials to the cells and carrying away wastes. The tubes—arteries, veins, and capillaries—reach every region of the body so that every cell receives nourishment.

The process of digestion produces nutrients in the form of food molecules, salts, vitamins, minerals, water, and oxygen. In the process of absorption, they enter the bloodstream to be transported to individual cells where they are converted to use according to the cell type or need. For example, in certain liver cells, the nutrients would be used to make the bile needed for proper digestion of fats. In the marrow of the body's long bones, nutrients would be used to make blood cells. In muscle tissue, the nutrients might be used for energy or to repair cells. In the skin, they would be used to make new skin cells to replace those that die. Every living cell needs the nutrients to do its work. Cells utilize nutrients though the process of metabolism—the fourth process in the conversion of food to function.

METABOLISM

Metabolism is the chemical process by which nutrients are transformed for use by the body's cells.

Cells are miniature factories that even produce their own energy. To do their work, they need the nutrients carried in the bloodstream. Living body cells are bathed by a liquid that comes from tiny nearby capillaries. Nutrients in the liquid pass through the cells' thin walls. Once inside the cells, they are used, or metabolized, to produce energy, make new tissue, or perform some other special function.

Nutrition is the combination of the separate but connected processes of digestion, absorption, circulation, and metabolism that move food, change it into usable forms, and then utilize it to maintain health. But the processes are only a part of how nutrition is linked to health and disease. For the processes to work, they need food in usable forms, that is, as nutrients.

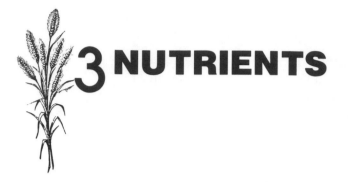

3 NUTRIENTS

Nutrients are substances in food that the body uses to maintain health. There are six classes of nutrients: carbohydrates, fats, proteins, vitamins, minerals, and water. They provide heat and energy, supply raw materials for tissue growth and repair, and help to regulate body processes.

A person's diet must contain various amounts of all the nutrients to maintain life and health, although different people require different amounts, depending on individual genetic and physiological differences. Although each nutrient has its own use, nutrients must work together. One cannot work unless others are present.

A person's age, sex, and size influence how much of each nutrient is required. Nutrient requirements are also affected by the person's environment and activity level. Someone lying in the sun on a beach on a summer day in California does not have to eat as much as a person chopping wood on a cold winter day in Alaska.

A principal function of nutrients is to supply the body with energy for warmth and work. Food energy is measured in calories, a unit of heat. One calorie is the amount of heat needed to raise the temperature of one gram of water one degree Celsius.

High-energy value foods are high in calories; low-energy value foods are low in calories. Fats have high-energy value and produce about nine calories per gram when burned. Carbohydrates and proteins produce about four calories per gram when they are burned.

Virtually all common foods have been measured for their calorie content, and the results can be found in books and lists called "calorie counters." The amount of calories burned by the body in performing various activities has also been calculated. For example, a person running at 10 miles per hour (16 kph) for an hour would burn approximately 900 calories, which is the amount available in eight to ten homemade brownies or fifteen slices of whole wheat bread. Playing the piano for an hour would burn only about 150 calories.

CARBOHYDRATES

Carbohydrates are the body's main source of energy and the most important class of nutrient in terms of amounts eaten. If the water and fiber in food were removed from one's diet, almost all of the rest would be carbohydrates. An average diet contains about 10 ounces (283.5 g) of carbohydrates for each ounce (28.35 g) of protein. Although the exact percentage of calories derived from carbohydrates in the American diet is disputed, the range is estimated to be from 40 to 55 percent of the calories. Carbohydrates are involved in virtually all of the body's many processes and functions, from making heat and moving muscles to digesting food and thinking. Most are used to produce the energy on which all metabolism depends. In a real sense, the body runs on carbohydrates in much the same way that a car runs on its fuel.

Carbohydrates are composed of carbon (carbo = carbon) and water (hydrate = combined with water). They are produced by plants in a process called photosynthesis, which, using the energy provided by sunlight, combines carbon dioxide from the air and water from the soil. When plants are eaten and metabolized, carbohydrates are "burned" (oxidized) by recombining with oxygen that is carried to the cells in the bloodstream. The process releases the energy locked in the carbohydrates. The energy is then used by the body for heat and work. The original materials used by plants to make carbohydrates, carbon dioxide, and water are also released.

A number of diseases, including diabetes, heart disease, high blood pressure, anemia, kidney problems, and cancer (some researchers add allergies and hyperactivity), may be linked with diets excessively high in refined carbohydrates. A refined carbohydrate is one from which some or all the nutrients other than carbohydrates have been removed. Everyday table sugar, for example, has had all of its associated nutrients removed.

Most carbohydrates found in food can be put into three major groups—sugars, starches, and cellulose. Sugars and starches are the body's principal energy sources. Most cellulose is indigestible and therefore supplies very little energy. Its bulk aids digestion and elimination. Sugars and starches are metabolized into simple sugars, mainly glucose, "blood sugar," the body's primary fuel.

Sugars, like the simple sugars contained in honey and fruit or more complex sugars like refined table sugar, are fairly easy to digest. Starches first must be broken down into simple sugars before they can be digested.

Glucose may be used immediately by the brain, nervous system, or body tissue after conversion from food, or it may go to the liver. The liver converts some excess glucose to glycogen, which is stored in the liver and in muscle tissue for later use. Most excess glucose is converted to fat, which is also stored. Stored glycogen is converted back to glucose when needed; stored fat is used directly.

FATS

From 40 to 45 percent of the calories in the American diet comes from the class of nutrients called fats. Fat, the body's most concentrated source of energy, supplies over twice the calories of an equal weight of carbohydrates or proteins. A gram of fat yields about nine calories while a gram of protein or carbohydrate yields about four.

Fats supply energy and essential fatty acids, aid in the transport of fat-soluble vitamins, and slow down digestion so that you feel full longer after eating foods containing fats. The heart, kidneys, and liver are protected by a covering of stored fat. Stored fat also insulates the body and helps to keep it warm. A layer of fat beneath the skin helps to smooth the body's shape by filling in the space between the muscles and skin.

Dietary fats come from animals or vegetables and can be solid or liquid. Liquid fats are oils. Fats are made of fatty acids which can be either *saturated* or *unsaturated*. Most animal fat is saturated; most vegetable fat is unsaturated.

Saturated fats usually remain firm at room temperature. Unsaturated fats are usually liquid at room temperature. Unsaturated fats can be converted into solid form by adding hydrogen (hydrogenation). Margarine made by the hydrogenation of vegetable oil is an example. Unsaturated fatty acids are important to growth, the health of the circulatory and nervous systems, and healthy skin. They also are involved in the body's utilization of cholesterol.

Cholesterol
Cholesterol an alcohol, not a fat—is a waxy, fatlike substance naturally found in most body tissue, partic-

39

ularly in the brain, nervous system, and blood. It plays a role in a number of body processes. In digestion, for example, a form of cholesterol in bile helps to break down fats so they can be absorbed through the wall of the small intestine.

The body obtains a third of its cholesterol from food and makes the rest, mostly in the liver. A deficiency is rare, but excess cholesterol is common in people who eat lots of saturated fats. Excess cholesterol may also be an inherited condition. Excessive cholesterol in blood may lead to a variety of diseases, including cardiovascular disease. In cardiovascular disease, excess cholesterol attaches itself to the walls of the arteries to form hard deposits called arterial plaque. If the deposits grow thick enough, they can clog an artery so that only a small trickle of blood can pass through. The tissues that normally would be nourished by the nutrient- and oxygen-rich blood become starved. When this happens in the heart, a heart attack occurs.

However, a high-fat diet does not automatically lead to heart disease. For example, the Masai of Africa eat a diet high in meat, milk, and blood, but do not have the heart problems associated with the American diet. Neither do the Inuit, who ate their traditional very high-fat diet and did not have circulatory problems until switching to a Western-type diet. Heart specialists who operate on patients with heart disease find that from a third to a half have normal cholesterol levels.

A recent study in the United States of 65,000 children aged three to eighteen found that one in five had high blood cholesterol levels—levels over 200 mg/dl (milligrams per deciliter).[1] One-fourth to one-third of children in the United States are estimated to have levels above 176 mg/dl. Normal cholesterol levels for children are in the 140 to 170 mg/dl range.

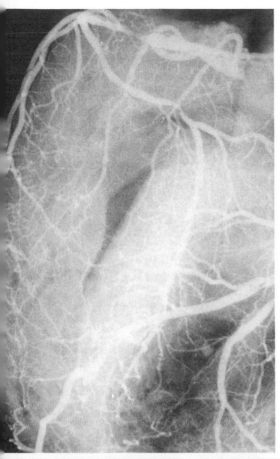

Left: *In this arteriogram of the human heart, obstructions in the arteries are plainly visible. These obstructions are due to the formation of fatty substances known as cholesterol.*

Below: *This patient in the cardiac intensive care unit of a hospital in Chicago is linked to machines that constantly monitor his vital signs.*

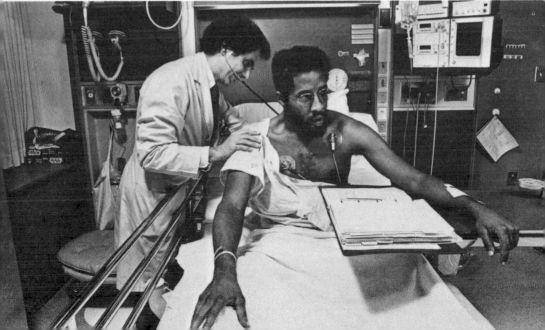

PROTEIN

Protein, the third class of nutrients, is the stuff the body is "made" of. Protein is made up of amino acids. The body manufactures all but eight or nine of the twenty to twenty-two amino acids an adult needs to make protein. The nine amino acids the body cannot make are called essential amino acids because they must come from the diet. All of the essential amino acids must be available at the same time or much of the body's production of protein will slow down or stop.

Complete protein foods contain all the essential amino acids necessary for protein synthesis in the body. Meat and dairy products are examples of complete protein foods.

Incomplete protein foods—nuts, seeds, grains, and most fruits and vegetables—do not supply all the required amino acids for making protein. Vegetarians who do not eat any animal products, for example, must mix a variety of incomplete protein foods to assure a combination that will supply all the essential amino acids. The problem is not as great for vegetarians who eat eggs and dairy products.

There is more protein in the body than any other substance except water (the average adult is 60 percent water). Muscles, blood, skin, hair, nails, the heart, the brain, and internal organs are mostly protein.

The amino acids obtained from protein in food are used for the formation of new proteins and tissues. The proteins help control growth, metabolism, sexual development, and water balance. The body can also burn protein for heat and energy, although it is the last substance used for this purpose if there are enough carbohydrates and fats available. A starving person or someone on a severely restricted diet will burn protein to survive, but the cost is valuable muscle tissue, including heart muscle. From 5 to 15 percent of the calories of the average American diet come from proteins. One study showed that the average protein intake in the United States is as much as 75 percent above the recommended dietary allowance (RDA) for men and 34 percent above the RDA for women.[2]

A deficiency of protein in the diet can lead to loss of energy, depression, weakness, unusual growth and tissue development, and poor muscle tone. It can also affect the growth of hair, nails, and skin and can reduce the body's resistance to infection, slow the healing of injuries, and impair recovery from illness.

VITAMINS

By the start of the twentieth century, scientists suspected there were unknown substances in foods that were essential to good health. The experiences with scurvy and its elimination by the addition of lime juice to British sailors' diets, the devastation by beriberi of Japanese sailing ship crews who ate polished rice, the rickets seen in children whose diets lacked vitamin D, and other examples showed that something more than carbohydrates, fats, and protein was needed in the diet.

Beriberi had puzzled scientists for years. In 1906 a British biochemist, Sir Frederick Gowland Hopkins, suggested there were substances in food that were essential to the body's health.[3] He called them "accessory nutrients." A few years later, Casimir Funk, a Polish biochemist, described a substance that he found prevented beriberi. He called his discovery a "vital amine" because it was a type of chemical known as an amine. The substance was thiamine (vitamin B_1), a material that is removed from rice when it is polished. Later the term for this and similar substances that were found necessary for a balanced diet became "vitamin," the name we use now for a whole class of important nutrients.

43

Vitamins are either water-soluble—they dissolve in water for transport to body tissues—or fat-soluble—they need dietary fats for transport. Water-soluble vitamins such as vitamin C and the B vitamins are measured in milligrams and micrograms. Fat-soluble vitamins like A, D, E, and K are measured in International Units (IUs) or United States Pharmacopoeia Units (USPs). Fat-soluble vitamins are stored in body fat and excessive levels can be dangerous. Water-soluble vitamins are easily excreted by the body so excess intake is not as likely to be harmful.

Vitamins are essential for good health and growth and must be obtained from sources outside the body—food or vitamin supplements. Generally, the body cannot make its own vitamins, though insufficient amounts of a few are produced by certain intestinal bacteria. No single food contains all the vitamins, so a variety of foods must be eaten to ensure a balanced diet.

Vitamins have a high level of biological activity—a little bit goes a long way. The small amounts present in the body are potent. They have no energy value and do not provide energy as carbohydrates do, and they do not combine with other nutrients to build tissue as protein does. They are parts of enzymes that break food down into basic elements for use by the body and help the enzymes act as catalysts. (Catalysts speed up or slow down chemical reactions without being changed themselves.)

There are fewer than twenty known vitamins, although there may be others that have not yet been discovered. Years of research on vitamins have led to the setting of "allowances" as a general guide to the nutritional needs of most healthy people. These Recommended Daily Allowances (RDAs) are recommendations by the Food and Nutrition Board of the National Academy of Sciences for average amounts of daily nutrient intake by healthy men, women, boys, and girls in different age groups. RDAs are not minimums; they are meant to exceed the *actual* daily requirement for individuals to maintain good health. The USRDAs—U.S. Recommended Daily Allowances—are a different set of guidelines. USRDAs are set by the U.S. Food and Drug Administration and represent the highest recommended daily allowance for each nutrient.[4] These are commonly listed on food labels.

Vitamin needs differ from one individual to another, and may change. A child may need more of a certain vitamin than an adult would; an adult who is ill may need more of one vitamin than a healthy adult would require. An individual's need for vitamins is influenced by age, health, heredity, exercise, personal habits such as smoking, and environmental factors such as pollution levels.

Vitamin deficiencies are not like infections or diseases that may appear suddenly. It can take weeks or months for signs of deficiency to be obvious. Like the poorly glowing bulb that does not get enough electricity to shine brightly, the body can continue to function with inadequate amounts of vitamins, but eventually the condition will become serious and may even result in death.

Vitamin A
Vitamin A is fat-soluble and is stored in the liver and kidneys. Natural sources of Vitamin A include carrots, tomatoes, eggs, spinach, parsley, winter squash, peaches, apricots, beef and fish liver, whole milk and milk products, and yellow and dark green fruits and vegetables.

Vitamin A is important for healthy skin, hair, mucous membranes, and body tissues. It is essential for good vision. Vitamin A also aids digestion by stimulating gastric juices.

45

Vitamin A may help prevent the development of a number of diseases and conditions, including asthma, emphysema, tuberculosis, glaucoma, migraine headaches, night blindness, measles, urogenital infections, the common cold, and some cancers.

The National Research Council's Recommended Dietary Allowance (RDA) is 1500 to 4000 International Units (IUs) for children and 4000 to 5000 IUs for adults. Individual needs may vary because of illness, environment, and general health. Too much vitamin A may lead to toxic effects such as nausea and vomiting, loss of appetite, hair loss, headaches, and diarrhea.

Vitamin B_1 (Thiamine)

Vitamin B_1 (and the other B-complex vitamins) is water-soluble and must be present in the diet daily because very little is stored in the body. It is found in whole wheat flour, yeast, wheat germ, whole grains, nuts, eggs, beef, pork, organ meats, fish, brown (unpolished) rice, beets, leafy green vegetables, and potatoes. Vitamin B_1 was the missing factor that caused beriberi in Japanese sailors and others whose diet was composed chiefly of polished rice.

Vitamin B_1 is quickly absorbed by the body and carried to the liver, heart, and kidneys, where it helps to make enzymes that aid in the metabolism of carbohydrates to simple sugars. Also called thiamine, this vitamin can be destroyed when exposed to air and heat outside the body. Smoking or consumption of alcohol, and refined sugar in the body, also increase the breakdown of vitamin B_1.

Vitamin B_1 is important for the conversion of carbohydrates into simple sugars the body can use. It also helps to stabilize the appetite by aiding in the digestion of sugars, starches, and alcohol.

Vitamin B_1 deficiency may lead to loss of appetite, fatigue, loss of mental alertness and emotional stability, memory loss, and gastrointestinal discomfort. Its importance to the central nervous system is due to its role in metabolizing carbohydrates to glucose.

The RDA for thiamine is 1.1 to 1.5 milligrams for children ages eleven to eighteen. It has no known toxicity.

Vitamin B₂ (Riboflavin)

Like other B-complex vitamins, vitamin B_2, or riboflavin, is water-soluble. It is found in brewer's yeast, liver, organ meats, whole grains, cheese, avocados, leafy green vegetables, egg yolks, blackstrap molasses, legumes, and nuts. Vitamin B_2 is readily absorbed in the small intestine. It helps in the metabolism of carbohydrates and the utilization of oxygen by the cells. Some vitamin B_2 is stored in the kidneys and liver, but regular amounts are needed to maintain adequate amounts in the system. Excess riboflavin is excreted in urine. A deficiency may lead to visual disturbances, light sensitivity, and eye fatigue.

Individual differences such as body size, growth rate, metabolic rate, and daily calorie intake may affect one's need for riboflavin. This vitamin may have a beneficial effect on vision problems.

The RDA for vitamin B_2 is 1.5 to 1.8 milligrams for males and 1.2 milligrams for females. B_2 has no known toxicity.

Vitamin B₃ (Niacin or Nicotinic Acid)

Vitamin B_3, niacin, is a part of the B-complex vitamin group and is water-soluble. Small quantities are found in foods including brewer's yeast, liver, turkey, tuna fish, chicken, whole wheat, lean meats, milk and milk products, eggs, rice bran, brown rice, and peanuts. It is not as susceptible to being broken down and destroyed by heat, light, oxidation, alkali, and acids as is vitamin B_2.

B_3 acts with other enzymes in the metabolism and

47

utilization of nutrients, including proteins, fats, and carbohydrates. The body is able to manufacture its own niacin by converting tryptophan, an amino acid that comes from outside sources.

Vitamin B_3 improves blood circulation, may aid in the reduction of cholesterol in the blood, assists the digestive process, and helps maintain the health of the skin and tongue. It is important to the proper functioning of the nervous system and is needed for the production of sex hormones. When administered to treat a deficiency, Vitamin B_3 may help to relieve migraine headaches, and improve nervous system function and the circulation to the extremities. Vitamin B_3 may also help to relieve high blood pressure and generally aid the circulation and digestion.

Indications that B_3 is lacking in the diet are bad breath, canker sores, irritability, nausea, and vomiting. There may also be loss of appetite, fatigue and muscular weakness, indigestion, and skin problems. Depression and recurring headaches have been associated with niacin deficiency.

Pellagra, a deficiency disease that is characterized by a rash on exposed body surfaces and sometimes by skin that looks badly sunburned, diarrhea, ulcers in the mouth, and depression or mental disorientation have been helped by the vitamin.

The RDA for vitamin B_3 is 6.6 grams per 1,000 calories, with 17 milligrams the suggested amount for men and 15 milligrams the amount suggested for women. The suggested RDA for children is 9 to 17 milligrams. Individual requirements vary according to growth needs, illness or injury, and level of physical activity.

Some doctors warn that very high doses of niacin (15,000 to 30,000 milligrams) may be dangerous, but it is not generally considered to have toxic effects. A large dose of 100 or more milligrams may produce a deep flushing of the skin caused by dilation of the blood vessels and a tingling, itching sensation and possible throbbing in the head which may last as long as 15 minutes. Long-term high-level intakes may produce liver damage and other problems.

Vitamin B₅ (Pantothenic Acid)

Vitamin B_5 (pantothenic acid), another of the water-soluble B-complex vitamins, is found in nearly all living cells—from one-celled organisms such as bacteria to the individual cells of all higher plants and animals. It is found in brewer's yeast, eggs, meat, wheat germ, crude molasses, whole-grain breads and cereals, legumes, and salmon. Naturally occurring bacteria in the intestines produce vitamin B_5.

Vitamin B_5 aids in cellular metabolism; helps to break down carbohydrates, fats, and proteins; helps to maintain a healthy digestive system; and may help the body to withstand stress. It is necessary for the production of cholesterol and fatty acids and stimulates the adrenal glands to produce adrenal hormones that are important to health.

A deficiency of vitamin B_5 is rare because it is so abundant. However, much of the vitamin may be lost when food is processed. When a deficiency occurs, reduced adrenal hormone production, low blood sugar, vomiting, abdominal pains, muscular cramps, and depression may occur.

There is no RDA for pantothenic acid and there are no known toxic effects.

Vitamin B₆ (Pyridoxine)

A water-soluble, B-complex vitamin, vitamin B_6 is not stored in the body in quantity. Vitamin B_6 is found in brewer's yeast, beef, brown rice, leafy green vegetables, wheat germ, bananas, walnuts, carrots, peanuts, milk and eggs, blackstrap molasses, and organ meats.

It is important for the metabolism of fats, carbohydrates, and proteins and aids in the absorption of vitamin B_{12}. It also aids in the production of hydrochloric acid, which is essential to digestion. Vitamin B_6 helps to regulate body fluid balance by regulating the body's sodium and potassium levels. It is also important to healthy red blood cells.

Hardening of the inner lining of the arteries (atherosclerosis) may be helped by vitamin B_6. It may help in the treatment of eczema (any inflammatory disease of the skin) and edema (the abnormal accumulation of water in the tissues) and in the treatment of stress.

It is a natural diuretic (a substance that stimulates the passage of urine).

Vitamin B_6 is normally excreted from the body within eight hours. A deficiency may be indicated by hair loss, cracks in the skin around the eyes and mouth, arm and leg cramps, and visual disturbances. Depression, irritability, nervousness, and muscular weakness may also indicate a deficiency.

The amount of vitamin B_6 needed daily is determined by how much protein is eaten. The National Research Council recommends 2 milligrams of vitamin B_6 per 100 grams of protein for adults, and up to 1.7 milligrams per 100 grams of protein for children as a daily requirement. Very large doses (2,000 to 6,000 milligrams daily) may cause serious nerve damage.

Vitamin B_9 (Folic Acid)
A water-soluble part of the B complex, vitamin B_9 (folic acid) is found in dark green leafy vegetables, broccoli, asparagus, peanuts, kidney and lima beans, wheat, organ meats, yeast, and whole-grain cereals. It is one of the few vitamins thought to be at low levels in the standard American diet. It plays a role in growth, increases the appetite, and is important for cellular reproduction.

The body needs folic acid to manufacture certain body proteins and genetic materials. It helps to prevent anemia (a condition characterized by low levels of hemoglobin, or red blood cells) and promotes the manufacture of hemoglobin, the blood protein that transports oxygen. It is needed for healthy hair and skin and may help to prevent premature graying of the hair. It also assists the body in producing the hydrochloric acid used in digestion.

Folic acid is destroyed by heat and light when stored for long periods at room temperature. Processing such as canning and extended cooking can also destroy the vitamin.

A deficiency may be indicated by anemia (reduced hemoglobin in the blood), inflammation of the tongue, prematurely graying hair, and gastrointestinal problems.

The RDA for folic acid is 150 to 200 micrograms. There is no known toxicity associated with excess folic acid.

Vitamin B_{12} (Cobalamin)

Vitamin B_{12}, a water-soluble B-complex vitamin, is obtained mainly from animal sources as it does not occur in other foods. It can be found in organ meats, clams, oysters and sardines, other fish and meats, egg yolks, and milk. Unlike many other vitamins, it cannot be artificially synthesized, but it is grown in molds, as is penicillin.

Vitamin B_{12} is important for proper carbohydrate, fat, and protein metabolism and is necessary for the utilization of some amino acids and vitamin C. It is important to nervous system metabolism, assists in the development of red blood cells, and helps the body to use iron.

Pernicious anemia, a form of anemia that affects mainly older people, results from the body's inability to absorb B_{12}. Some nervous system damage with

51

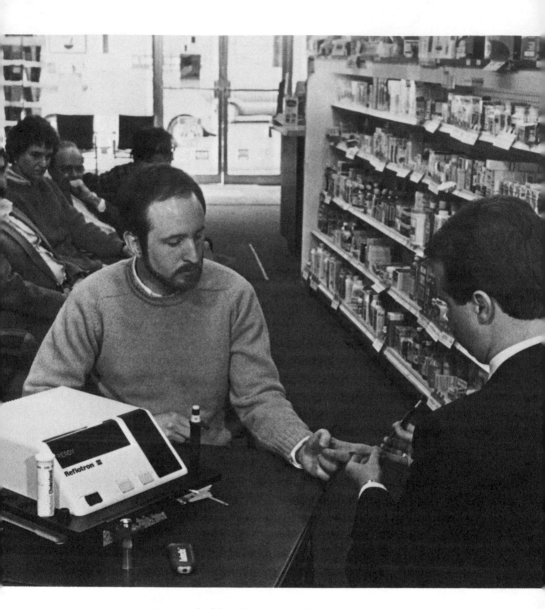

A simple blood test, such as the one given in this drugstore, can determine whether or not someone has anemia, a deficiency of hemoglobin in the blood.

symptoms such as reduced sensory perception, jerky limb movement, weak arms and legs, and difficulty in walking and speaking is also possible. Permanent mental and physical damage may result if a B_{12} deficiency, usually caused by failure to absorb the vitamin, is not corrected. Treatment for deficiencies of vitamin B_{12}, as with any other condition, should be by a physician.

Vitamin B_{12} may help restore mild memory loss and the ability to concentrate, relieve nervousness and insomnia, and aid in reducing depression and fatigue if they are due to inadequate intake.

Normal requirements for vitamin B_{12} are quite small. RDAs are 2 micrograms for adults. Growing children may need 1 to 2 micrograms. There are no known toxic effects from excesses of vitamin B_{12}.

Vitamin C (Ascorbic Acid)
Vitamin C is a well-known, water-soluble vitamin that plays a role in many body functions. Most animals manufacture their own vitamin C, but humans must obtain it from outside sources. The most abundant sources are citrus fruits, tomatoes, broccoli, cauliflower, sweet peppers, dark green leafy vegetables, melons, and strawberries.

A primary function of vitamin C is to help the body fight off infection. It also helps to protect other nutrients from oxidation. Formation of collagen, a protein essential for building the body's connective tissues, depends on vitamin C. Vitamin C also aids in the healing process and helps the body to overcome the effects of stress. It may be effective in treating allergies and viral and bacterial infections including the common cold.

Scurvy, a serious deficiency disease, results when the diet lacks vitamin C. Inadequate vitamin C may be the cause of poor digestion, anemia, reduced resistance to infection, swollen and painful joints, bleeding gums, nosebleeds, and easy bruising. A deficiency can also lead to the weakening of capillary walls, which in turn may lead to heart attacks and strokes caused by blood clots.

Vitamin C is flushed out of the body and must be replaced. It is excreted in the urine and most excess is out of the body within four hours. Stress, smoking, high fever, aspirin, and some pain killers impair the body's absorption of vitamin C. Extra amounts are needed during periods of stress, infection, and injury. The RDA for vitamin C is 60 milligrams for men and women. Smokers should consume 100 milligrams daily. Body weight, activity level, and metabolic rate may influence the need for the vitamin.

Very large amounts may produce toxic affects.

Vitamin D

Vitamin D is fat-soluble and so the body is able to store it. Most is stored in the liver. Natural sources of vitamin D include fish liver oils, salmon, herring and sardines, egg yolks, bone meal, organ meats, and vitamin D-fortified milk and milk products. Vitamin D is also synthesized in the body when the sun's ultraviolet rays strike the skin. Because dark skin blocks ultraviolet rays, people with dark complexions must obtain vitamin D from their diet.

Vitamin D helps to regulate the absorption of calcium and phosphorus and is essential for bone growth and repair. It is also important for healthy teeth.

Vitamin D deficiency affects the bones, skeleton, and teeth. Rickets, a disease of children characterized by bowed legs, funnel chest, and other bone deformities, is a serious vitamin D deficiency disease. Osteomalacia, an adult form of rickets in which the bones soften, is also a vitamin D deficiency disease.

The RDA for vitamin D is 400 IUs. Overdosing is

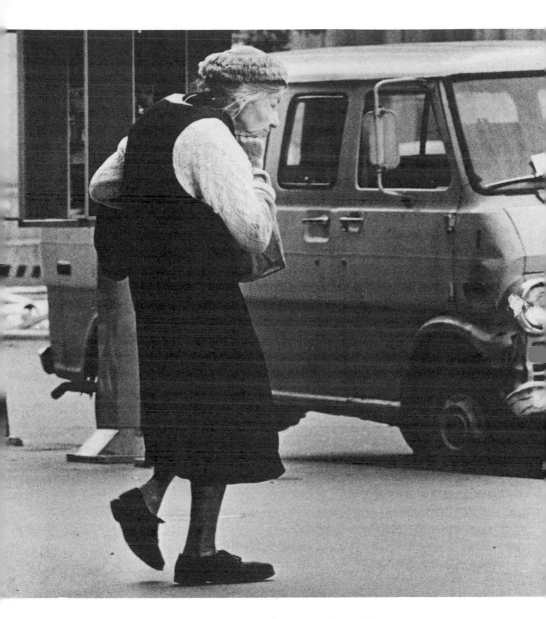

Osteoporosis, a disease that affects more women than men, results in deformed and fragile bones that are easily broken.

possible and can result in nausea, vomiting, dizziness, frequent urination, loss of appetite, diarrhea, and the deposit of calcium in body tissues such as the heart, lungs, and blood vessels. Some researchers warn that very high amounts for infants and children can be toxic.

Vitamin E
This vitamin differs from other fat-soluble vitamins in that the body stores it for relatively short periods of time only. Vitamin E is found naturally in vegetable oils such as safflower, sunflower, and soybean oils, and margarine, wheat germ, nuts, whole grains, molasses, dark green leafy vegetables, and sweet potatoes. Vitamin E is an anti-oxidant, which means that it prevents or inhibits oxygen from combining with other substances. Oxidation in the body can be harmful. For example, some of the effects of aging are the result of oxidation in body cells. Vitamin E acts to prevent this.

Vitamin E aids circulation by slowing the formation of cholesterol plaque. It aids in the healing of scratches and burns and reduces the formation of scar tissue. Vitamin E's anti-oxidant effect allows cells to utilize other vitamins, minerals, and hormones more effectively.

A deficiency of vitamin E is rare. The amount of vitamin E needed depends on a person's metabolism. Because vitamin E raises the blood pressure and large doses may lead to dangerous blood clots, this vitamin should be used with caution. The RDAs for vitamin E are 12 IUs for males aged eleven to fourteen years and 15 IUs for men fifteen years and older. For all women from age eleven up, the RDA is 12 IUs.

Vitamin K
Natural vitamin K is produced in the intestinal tract. It also is found in cow's milk, kelp, leafy green vege-

tables, cabbage, cauliflower, peas, yogurt, fish liver oils, safflower and soybean oils, egg yolks, and meat. It is a fat-soluble vitamin.

Vitamin K plays a role in blood clotting. It is needed to prevent nosebleeds, bruising, and excessive bleeding from cuts or scratches. Vitamin K also aids in the conversion of glucose into glycogen, the form of sugar that is stored in the liver for use as fuel, when needed, by other parts of the body. It is important for the normal function of the liver.

The 1989 RDAs for vitamin K range from 5 micrograms per day for a newborn to a high of 80 micrograms per day for an adult male. Natural vitamin K is not known to cause toxic reactions.

MINERALS

Minerals constitute another class of nutrients. The minerals in foods originate in the earth. In the soil in microscopic forms (mineral crystals) that dissolve in water, they are first utilized by plants, which take them up and incorporate them in vegetable matter. They are passed on to animals, including humans, when the plants are eaten. About 4 to 5 percent of the weight of the human body is mineral matter.

There are about seventeen minerals that are essential to human nutrition. They can be found in all body tissues and fluids in varying, very small amounts. Bones and teeth, muscles, blood, and nerve tissues are partly made of minerals. Minerals work in conjunction with the vitamins. They give strength to the skeleton, aid physiological processes, and act as catalysts in muscle action, the transmission of nerve impulses, digestion, and metabolism. They are also helpful in maintaining the body's water balance and acid-alkali balance. Like the vitamins, minerals work in unison. The effects of one affect the others.

The major minerals or macronutrients—calcium, chlorine, phosphorus, potassium, magnesium, sodium, and sulfur—are relatively abundant in the body. Others, known as "trace minerals," or micronutrients, are present in extremely small amounts. All minerals are important.

Mineral deficiencies are not common for those who eat a wide variety of foods. However, many people do not get all the minerals they need, particularly teenagers who are dieting or not varying their diets. It is best to regulate mineral intake through the diet rather than by taking supplements.[5]

Calcium

Calcium, the body's most abundant mineral, is necessary for the growth of bones, teeth, and muscle tissue. Sources of calcium are milk and milk products (yogurt, cheeses, ice cream), canned salmon (with the bones), citrus fruits, peas, beans, soybeans, peanuts, sunflower seeds, leafy dark green vegetables, kidney beans, clams, oysters, and shrimp. Calcium aids in metabolism and regulates muscle contraction and expansion, including the heartbeat. It is important for nerve function and the clotting of blood. Almost all calcium in the body (99 percent, or about 2 to 3 pounds) is in the bones and teeth.

A deficiency may result in poor growth, muscle and nerve sensitivity, heart palpitations, high blood pressure, fragile bones, muscle cramps, and painful joints.

The RDA for calcium ranges from 400 milligrams per day for a newborn to a high of 1,200 milligrams a day for young adults.

Chlorine

Chlorine is found in the body combined as chloride with sodium or potassium. In the normal diet it comes from table salt, but is also found in kelp, cabbage, celery, oats, watercress, pineapple, and tomatoes. It is essential for the synthesis of hydrochloric acid, an important component of digestive juices, and aids liver function and helps to regulate the body's acid-alkali balance.

Excess chloride normally is excreted from the body through sweating. A deficiency may result in hair or tooth loss, poor digestion of fibrous foods, and poor muscle contraction.

Chromium

The effects of chromium on body functions are important even though there is very little of this essential mineral in the body. Chromium is found in brewer's yeast, meat, mushrooms, cheese, corn and corn oil, shellfish, and whole grains. Chromium is especially important in the metabolism and transport of glucose. It also helps to prevent high blood pressure.

Chromium deficiencies may be associated with the refinement of foods that strips away this and other important nutrients. There is no RDA for chromium, but nutritionists believe many people get substantially less than the desirable amount.

Copper

Copper is found in very small amounts in the body where it is important for nerve function, skin and hair pigmentation, bone growth and health, protein metabolism, and the oxidation of vitamin C. It also aids in the manufacture of red blood cells. Sources of copper are calf and beef liver, dried beans, peas, shrimp, oysters, most seafood, nuts, and fruits.

A deficiency may result in anemia, edema, skin problems, fatigue, and osteoporosis (loss of bone mass). There is no RDA for copper. Excessive amounts of copper may be toxic.

Fluorine

Fluorine is found in bones and teeth and is helpful in preventing tooth decay. It also helps to strengthen bones. Sources include fluoridated water supplies, seafood, cheese, milk, cereal grains, animal products, and dental products.

Excessive amounts of this essential mineral may be harmful. Too much fluorine may affect the metabolism of vitamins and may harm the kidneys, liver, heart, and central nervous system. Tooth decay may result from a deficiency.

There is no RDA for fluorine.

Iodine

One-third of the body's iodine, a trace mineral important for the proper functioning of the thyroid gland, is found in that gland, which is located in the neck. The thyroid helps to control metabolism. Excellent sources of iodine are saltwater fish and seafood, kelp, sea salt, iodized salt, garlic, pears, mushrooms, and pineapples.

Iodine deficiencies are rare in the United States but quite common in other areas. A deficiency may cause poor metabolism, hardening of the arteries, sluggish mental activity, heart palpitations, and nervousness. Goiter, an enlargement of the thyroid gland, is a sign of iodine deficiency.

The RDA for iodine is 150 micrograms for adults. There are no known toxic effects from naturally occurring iodine, but large amounts may seriously affect the thyroid gland.

Iron

Iron is found in the body combined with protein. Liver, sardines, oysters, brewer's yeast, lentils, prunes and raisins, dark green leafy vegetables, eggs, whole-grain cereals, and lean meat are sources of iron. Copper and calcium must be present in the body for iron to work effectively. Iron is important in the manufacture of hemoglobin, the blood protein that carries oxygen to the cells of the body. Iron is also important in helping the body reduce susceptibility to stress and disease. It can help to prevent depression, fatigue, weakness, headaches, and poor concentration. It also plays a role in muscle function.

Low iron in the body may cause iron-deficiency anemia, the most common worldwide nutritional deficiency.[6] In the United States, iron deficiency is common among teenage girls and women, affecting about one out of four. About 5 percent suffer anemia. Women lose twice as much iron as men, because of blood loss during menstruation. Symptoms are unusual fatigue, sickly looking skin, constipation, brittle nails, and difficulty breathing.

Iron is stored in the liver, blood, spleen, and bone marrow and is used over and over. The RDAs for iron are 10 milligrams daily for men and 15 milligrams daily for women. Excessive iron may damage the liver, induce a deficiency of vitamin C, and cause the skin to turn metallic gray.

Magnesium
Magnesium is an essential mineral important for carbohydrate and mineral metabolism, muscle function, bone growth, acid-alkali balance, and the utilization of glucose for energy. Dietary magnesium is found in soybeans, raw wheat germ, green vegetables, figs, lemons, grapefruit, corn, apples, nuts, seeds, whole grains, and shellfish. Magnesium aids in the transmission of nerve impulses and helps the body deal with physical and emotional stress.

A magnesium deficiency may result in heart disease, blood clots in the heart and brain, muscle tremors, confusion, and disorientation.[7] Excess magnesium in the diet may lead to drowsiness, lethargy, stupor, and coma. People with heart or kidney conditions should consult a doctor before taking magnesium supplements.

The RDA for magnesium is 270 to 400 milligrams for males and 280 to 300 milligrams for females. It is estimated that the average American gets only about three-fourths of the magnesium recommended for good health.

Manganese

Manganese is present in trace quantities in the body and works in conjunction with other substances as a catalyst in the utilization of B vitamins and vitamin C. Manganese is obtained from nuts, whole-grain cereals, wheat germ, spinach, grapefruit, oranges, and green vegetables. Manganese aids in the manufacture of sex hormones and milk, and plays a role in the production of fatty acids and cholesterol. It is important for skeletal growth.

The ability of the body to remove excess sugar from the blood may be affected by a deficiency of manganese. Poor muscle coordination also may be a deficiency sign. Other symptoms of deficiency include noises in the ears, hearing loss, and dizziness.

Manganese may be helpful in treating diabetes, and loss of muscle coordination and strength, and some researchers think it may be useful in treating multiple sclerosis, an auto-immune disease.

There is no RDA for manganese. The average diet supplies an adequate amount.

Phosphorus

Phosphorus is abundant in the body and is present in every cell. Phosphorus is found in high-protein foods such as fish, meat, poultry, and eggs, and in whole grains, dried fruits, and corn. Phosphorus is believed to play a role in virtually all the body's chemical reactions. It is involved in the use of proteins, fats, and carbohydrates for growth, repair, and energy supply. It is essential for bone development and helps muscle contraction. It also aids appetite control. It is necessary for healing and glandular activity, and may help in keeping the mind alert.

Phosphorus deficiency does not occur among healthy people. A deficiency may result in poor bone and tooth growth and rickets, and may be a factor in arthritis. Weakness, loss of appetite, listlessness, and bone pain are also signs of phosphorus deficiency.

The RDA for phosphorus is 800 to 1,200 milligrams. Experts sometimes suggest calcium be taken with phosphorus in the same amounts as they work together in the body. Excess phosphorus can produce hypocalcemic tetany, a serious muscular condition.

Potassium

Potassium is important for every body function. Vegetables, bananas, potatoes, dates, raisins, apricots, cantaloupe, oranges and orange juice, prune juice, turkey, tomatoes, broccoli, whole-grain cereals, sunflower seeds, and nuts are sources of potassium. Potassium is vital to normal metabolism and growth. It works to maintain fluid balance and the acid-alkali balance in the body. With other substances, it aids the conversion of glucose to glycogen for storage in the liver. It helps to maintain a regular heartbeat and is important for the transport of oxygen to the brain. It aids in maintaining healthy skin and is also an aid to proper elimination.

Nerve disorders, irregular heartbeat, overall weakness, poor reflexes, dry skin, saggy muscles, and nausea and dizziness after excessive sweating are some of the signs of potassium deficiency.

There is no RDA for potassium, although some experts recommend 1,600 to 3,500 milligrams daily

63

for adults. The normal diet supplies from 2,000 to 6,000 milligrams.

There are no toxic effects known from potassium.

Selenium

Like vitamin E, selenium, an essential mineral that is present in small quantities in the body, acts as an antioxidant, is involved in a number of metabolic functions, aids growth, and helps prevent aging. Sources for this mineral include bran, yeast, seafood, meat, liver, kidneys, radishes, eggs, mushrooms, wheat germ, and milk.

Selenium deficiency, perhaps in conjunction with a virus, is thought to be responsible for Keshan disease, a form of heart disease observed in some areas of China. No similar deficiency has been reported in the United States. A number of studies have correlated low blood levels of selenium with a high cancer risk.[8]

The body requires only small amounts of selenium. The RDA is 40 to 70 micrograms for males and 45 to 55 micrograms for females. Excess amounts may produce a metallic taste in the mouth, dizziness, unexplained lethargy, progressive paralysis, and fragile or black fingernails. Selenium poisoning can be fatal.

Sodium

Sodium is an essential mineral that works with potassium to maintain the blood's acid-alkali balance and in cellular functions. With potassium, sodium helps muscle activity and aids in maintaining the body's proper water balance. Sodium is present in most foods, especially processed foods, seafood, meat, poultry, bacon, organ meats, table salt, and sometimes in water, depending on its source.

Sodium is strongly linked to high blood pressure. An excess may also damage the kidneys and heart.

A sodium deficiency is rare because this mineral

is present in so many foods. Most people eat more sodium than is necessary for health. There is no RDA for sodium, but experts suggest keeping the intake as low as possible.

Sulfur

Sulfur helps the body maintain youthful looking skin and smooth, glossy hair. It works with other substances to help in the metabolism of carbohydrates, aids in the production of collagen, and helps to build body tissue. Sulfur is found in fish, nuts, radishes, meat, eggs, cabbage, brussels sprouts, soybeans, and dried beans.

Deficiency signs may include sluggishness and fatigue. There is no RDA for sulfur. Excess sulfur may be toxic.

Zinc

Zinc is found in very small quantities in the body. Zinc is associated with a number of enzymes that aid digestion and metabolism. It is essential for growth and is important to the development of the reproductive system. Zinc aids the formation of insulin, helps regulate muscle contractions, and aids in protein metabolism. It is important to a healthy immune system. Sources of zinc include brewer's yeast, wheat germ, sunflower seeds, wheat bran, eggs, lamb, liver, poultry, whole grains, non-fat dry milk, and seafood.

A zinc deficiency may produce retarded growth, slow wound healing, white spots on the fingernails, rashes, mental dullness, difficulty concentrating, and increased susceptibility to infections.

The RDA for zinc is 12 milligrams daily for females and 15 milligrams daily for males. The average diet contains from 10 to 15 milligrams of zinc. Excess zinc in the diet may produce vomiting, diarrhea, drowsiness, and anemia.

Amino Acids

Amino acids are the building blocks of protein molecules (see page 42). Protein molecules in food are broken down in the body into amino acids, which are then used to build the body's own proteins.

Amino acids are still not fully understood. It is not certain exactly how many there are; there are believed to be about twenty. It is known that they are essential in human nutrition. Their effects in the body include the alleviation of chronic pain, the stabilization of energy swings, the control of kidney failure, the relief of arthritis, and the reduction of the appetite. They are involved in the synthesis of proteins that help carry oxygen to tissues and cells, aid in the manufacture of hormones, help digestion, and even aid the process of thinking.

The body makes many of its own amino acids, but others, the essential amino acids, must come from the diet. All amino acids are necessary for good health.

PLANNING A GOOD DIET

There is probably no ideal diet that would be right for everyone. But despite the many physical differences among people, and differences in their ways of life, everyone needs all nutrients, although varying amounts of each nutrient may be required. Also, there is no ideal food that contains all the nutrients needed for complete nutrition. To get all the necessary nutrients for good health a person has to eat a wide variety of foods grown in different regions.

In 1956, the United States Department of Agriculture established dietary guidelines based on "food groups"—grains, fruits and vegetables, meat, and dairy products. Eating a selection of foods from each group assured a balanced diet, that is, a diet that contained all the nutrients required for good health. The concept of basic food groups is now being challenged by scientists, nutritionists, and others who are concerned about the demonstrated effects of diet on health. For example, diseases such as cancer and heart disease have increased greatly in countries that have changed from traditional diets consisting primarily of grains, fish, and vegetables to the typical, high-fat American diet heavy in meat and dairy products. It is now believed that a healthy diet should include more fruits, vegetables, and whole grains, and less meat and dairy foods.

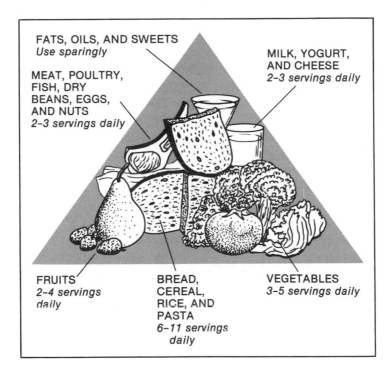

FATS, OILS, AND SWEETS
Use sparingly

MEAT, POULTRY, FISH, DRY BEANS, EGGS, AND NUTS
2–3 servings daily

MILK, YOGURT, AND CHEESE
2–3 servings daily

FRUITS
2–4 servings daily

BREAD, CEREAL, RICE, AND PASTA
6–11 servings daily

VEGETABLES
3–5 servings daily

Recent nutrition findings suggest that the typical, high-fat American diet should be replaced by this new food grouping.

New guidelines recommended by the Physicians Committee for Responsible Medicine keep the food groups, but rearrange them in a pyramid in order of their importance to a healthy diet from the bottom to the top. Breads and cereals are at the base (six to eleven servings daily), fruits (two to four servings) and vegetables (three to five servings) are at the next tier, meat (two to three servings) and dairy products (two to three servings) are at the level above that, and finally, at the top, are fats, oils, and sugars, which are to be eaten sparingly.

The National Research Council's Committee on Diet and Health recommends eating five or more servings of vegetables and fruits daily, eating a moderate amount of protein, reducing fat intake to 30 percent or less of the total calories consumed, limiting salt intake to 6 grams or less, consuming adequate amounts of calcium, avoiding alcohol and dietary supplements over RDA levels, drinking fluoridated water, and balancing food consumption with physical exercise to maintain an appropriate weight.

THE FOUR BASIC FOOD GROUPS

Grains (Breads and Cereals)
Foods in the grain group supply carbohydrates and some protein and iron, thiamin, and niacin. The group includes whole-grain and enriched breads, cereals, spaghetti and other forms of noodles, rice, barley and other grains, cracked wheat, cornmeal, and foods made with grain flour such as pancakes, waffles, muffins, and rolls.

Fruits and Vegetables
Fruits and vegetables are sources of vitamins A, B_2, B_6, C, folic acid, iron, magnesium and potassium, car-

bohydrates, and dietary fiber. They include apples, asparagus, bananas, berries, broccoli, brussels sprouts, cabbage, cantaloupe, carrots, cauliflower, chard, citrus fruits, collards, corn, green beans, kale, parsley, peaches, pears, peas, peppers, potatoes, raisins, red leaf lettuce, romaine lettuce, scallions, spinach, tomatoes, turnip greens, watercress, and more.

Meat

The word meat is often used as a convenient name for this food group that includes meat and meat products as well as other foods that supply substantial amounts of protein and iron and vitamins B_6 and B_{12}. Other foods in the group include poultry, eggs, seafood and fish, dried beans and peas, lentils, soybeans and soy products, peanuts, peanut butter, seeds, and nuts.

Dairy

Milk and milk products such as yogurt, cheese, cottage cheese, kefir, and ice cream are excellent sources of protein and calcium. They also supply vitamins A, B_2, and B_{12}. Fortified milk supplies vitamin D, and cheese is a source of zinc.

Fats and Sugars

Fats and oils, though not a separate food group, are important to the diet to supply energy, essential fatty acids, and some vitamin E. Butter, margarine, vegetable oil, cream, nuts, seeds, avocados, and olives are common sources. Fat consumption should be kept under 30 percent of daily calories.

Sugars and sweets—from jelly, candy, syrups, soft drinks, and bakery products—furnish calories and have some energy value.

Our understanding of nutrition is incomplete. While the importance of proper nutrition to good health is unquestionable, the complexity of the human body, the variety of materials it needs to function, and the knowledge that there is so much remaining to be discovered leave gaps in any discussion of the subject. Those gaps are being investigated and filled by researchers. Even with these uncertainties, fundamentals of nutrition demonstrate how deeply dependent the body is on its food supply.

PART III
NUTRITION
AND DISEASE

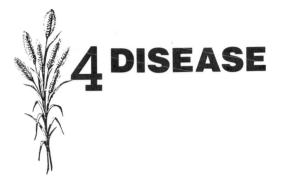

4 DISEASE

Starvation provides the most obvious and dramatic evidence that food and health are linked. For most of human history, the effects of starvation were the only connections that were understood between nutrition and disease. If you didn't eat, you got sick and died. It was as simple as that. The discoveries that linked specific diseases with specific nutrition deficiencies were not made until relatively recently.[1]

DEFICIENCY DISEASES

About 200 years ago James Lind found that citrus juice could prevent and cure scurvy. A Polish biochemist, Casimir Funk, discovered in 1910 that something important to human health—the "anti-beriberi factor" (vitamin B_1)—was removed when rice was milled. The first vitamins were identified and the theory of vitamin deficiency diseases was developed by scientists early in this century. Most deficiency diseases—rickets, pellagra, scurvy, beriberi, xerophthalmia (drying of the mucous membranes of the eye due to vitamin A deficiency) and goiter—were common throughout the United States and the world as recently as the 1940s. The links between nutrition and more complex diseases such as cancer, coronary heart disease, high blood pressure, and others are only now beginning to be understood.

Science's investigation of the relationship between nutrition and health is well under way, but far from complete. Our brief look at nutrition and body systems shows how the complexity of the human organism and the intricate chemistry of food can lead to more questions than answers. When many variables interact, thousands of associations are possible.

The early and easier questions were answered once the connection was made between certain nutrients and diseases. When it was realized that a lack in the diet was the cause of a disease, the missing nutrient was restored and the disease was eliminated. Vitamin D was added to milk to end the common childhood bone disease, rickets. Iodine added to salt (iodized salt) ended the thyroid condition called goiter. Other diseases were similarly eliminated so that today deficiency diseases are extremely rare in the United States.

OVER-NUTRITION DISEASES

Now researchers are investigating a different kind of disease-nutrition connection. It has to do with excess rather than deficiency. Over-nutrition and imbalanced diets—too much food and too much of the wrong kinds of food—are thought to play a significant part in five of the ten leading causes of illness and death in the country. They are heart disease, certain cancers, strokes, diabetes, and atherosclerosis. In addition, over-nutrition and dietary imbalances contribute to high blood pressure, obesity, dental diseases, osteoporosis, and gastrointestinal diseases.

Life has become considerably more complex since the early hunter-gatherers got their nutrition straight from nature's cupboard. And the immense body of knowledge we have built up in all fields of scientific and social inquiry has added to the complexity and made the uncovering of causes and effects more difficult. Someone looking for a nutrition-disease link a hundred years ago had to contend only with an observed problem—the symptoms of scurvy, for example—and the results of treatment—the disappearance of the symptoms after providing citrus juice. Today the problems we are looking at are much more complicated. We know that the environment, social conditions, and individual behavior and genetic differences all affect life and health. It is hard to find direct connections and simple conclusions.

Because of the many factors that can affect health, there is not always a directly observable connection between a disease and excessive or imbalanced nutrition. If two people eat an identical diet, one may suffer heart disease but not diabetes, and the other may suffer diabetes but not heart disease. Of course, neither may suffer anything at all and remain perfectly healthy while a third person on the same diet has a stroke. Or all three may remain disease-free while a fourth is diagnosed with cancer. Diet alone does not determine why some become ill while others thrive. Other factors contribute too—such as smoking, family medical history, workplace conditions, level of physical activity, and much more. Diet is a significant factor, but so are all other aspects of a person's life.

With so many nutritional and other factors affecting health, and because we are looking at a huge population, spread over a large area, it is difficult to gather precise information. It was easy to come to a conclusion about a disease affecting a ship's crew because they were few in number and all in one place. When, after a few months at sea, most showed the signs of scurvy, and when, on later voyages, the signs never appeared after citrus juice was included in the diet, the obvious and correct conclusion was that something in the juice prevented scurvy. Direct observation of large, spread-out populations is impractical. Today scientific conclusions about nutrition and disease are drawn from clinical studies of small groups, from animal studies, and from inferences drawn from indirect sources such as statistical studies.

With so many variables and indirect information that can be interpreted in different ways, we often are faced with differing opinions about nutrition and health. There is also much uncertainty. When the link between nutrition and diseases is not direct and easily visible, the conclusions about the link will be weaker than when there is an obviously direct cause-effect relationship. We are sometimes offered only "best guesses" and other times are faced with conflicting claims.

Fortunately, there is ample evidence from a variety of sources to allow reaching some firm—if not absolute—conclusions about the relationship of diet to health in general, and to a number of diseases in particular.

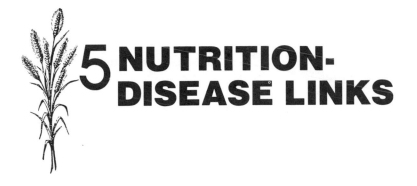

5 NUTRITION- DISEASE LINKS

"You are what you eat" is an overstatement if applied to the connection between diet and disease because many other factors influence life and health. Yet there is no question that nutrition plays a primary role in well-being. Overall nutrition affects your general health—a balanced diet will produce generally good health, and individual differences in diet affect specific areas of health—the lack of a necessary nutrient can produce disease.

ANEMIA

One of the principle functions of the circulatory system is to delivery oxygen from the lungs to the cells, where it is used to produce energy. The substance in the blood that carries oxygen is hemoglobin, a complex iron-protein compound. Anemia is a condition that occurs when there is too little hemoglobin in the blood, often caused by iron deficiency.

Iron deficiency persists in many less developed areas of the world and is still of some concern in the United States.

From about 1500 to 1900, young women often suffered from a form of iron deficiency called chlorosis. Its cause was not understood, though imaginative diagnoses included "lovesickness" and tight corsets. Victims were pale, breathless, and weak. In the early period, the condition was treated by bloodletting, a primitive medical treatment for numerous ailments and diseases in which patients were bled, sometimes to the point of death.

It took two hundred years for science and medicine to learn that iron was an important constituent of blood and that iron deficiency was linked to nutrition. In the 1680s the chemical composition of blood was analyzed for the first time. An English physician, Thomas Sydenham, began treating his anemic patients with a concoction made by steeping iron filings in wine, and found that their conditions improved. Two centuries later, iron was recognized to be an essential nutrient for animals and was one of the first substances identified as essential for the human diet. In 1926 physicians found they could cure anemia with an extract made from liver, which is high in iron as well as vitamin B_{12}.

Once it was clear that an iron-deficient diet was a cause of anemia, foods fortified with iron were introduced, and the rates of iron deficiency rapidly declined. Iron was added to cereal, flour, and grain products in the 1940s and to infant cereals and formulas in the 1950s. Although chlorosis vanished early in this century and the rates of iron deficiency disease have declined rapidly, awareness of the dangers of iron deficiency is essential.

The amount of iron in the body of an adult male is less than the weight of a nickel, but its role in oxygen transport makes this small amount of mineral essential to health.

Most iron is found in the hemoglobin or is stored in the liver, spleen, and bone marrow. Stored iron is used, along with iron taken in as part of the diet, to replace the small amounts that are normally lost daily through elimination, sweating, loss of cells, and bleeding.

Most iron in the body is used over and over and very little is lost (except in bleeding). But if the amount of iron lost is not replaced, a deficiency may result. People with greater stored reserves of iron are less likely to suffer iron deficiency than those whose reserves are low.

The need for dietary iron is greatest in young people. Infants being fed cow's milk (a poor source of iron), children and adolescents, and women of childbearing age are at the highest risk of iron deficiency.

Iron deficiency in adolescence is common, particularly during the years of sudden growth. Boys between the ages of twelve and fifteen may add twenty-two pounds in weight during peak growth; girls between ten and fifteen may add twenty pounds. For girls, blood loss through menstruation increases the need for dietary iron.

By eating a normal diet, adult men can easily replace the tiny amount of iron lost daily, but the high-risk groups for anemia require proportionately more iron in their diets. Women who experience greater than normal blood loss through menstruation and women who are pregnant are at particularly high risk. (About 20 percent of women have heavier than normal menstrual blood loss, but are unaware that their monthly loss is above average.)

Iron deficiency reduces the delivery of oxygen to all parts of the body. When body cells don't get the oxygen they need to function, their efficiency is reduced. Fatigue, impaired brain function, and poor temperature control are among the problems caused by inefficient oxygenation of cells. The body is also less resistant to infection. Work and exercise performance are diminished substantially, and there is a growing body of evidence that behavior and intellectual performance are impaired by iron deficiency as well.

Even though iron is one of earth's most abundant elements and is found in many foods, deficiencies can occur because it is not readily absorbed. Whole grains are an example of foods with iron that is not easily absorbed. They contain substantial amounts of iron, but in a form that does not dissolve easily.

It is believed that there is an adequate supply of iron in the average American diet to provide the required amounts of this essential mineral. However, the high-risk groups for anemia—infants, children, adolescents, and women of childbearing age—may need increased dietary iron.

The simplest way to add iron to the diet is through iron-rich foods. Supplements can provide added iron, but this is not usually recommended for the general population.

Absorption of iron can be increased by eating diets rich in meat, poultry, and fish and by adding foods and juices containing vitamin C to the diet. Coffee and tea reduce iron absorption.

ARTHRITIS

The term "arthritis" describes any inflammatory condition of skeletal joints that is characterized by pain and swelling. There are over a hundred forms of arthritis.[1] Arthritis is generally considered to be a common degenerative disease associated with aging, but it can occur at any age.

Affected joints are often those that bear weight, such as the hips, knees, and spine, but arthritis can affect any joint in the body where two bones come together. Most arthritis produces the same symptoms of pain, soreness, swelling, stiffness, and tenderness in the joints, often in the morning. The discomfort and restricted movement can make simple tasks such as walking and holding objects difficult or, in serious cases, impossible.

The exact causes of arthritis are not fully known. Some researchers believe the disease may be related to the body's immune system, which either does not produce enough antibodies to fight bacterial or viral infections in joints, or mistakes healthy cells for viruses and destroys both. Others link the inflammation of arthritis with allergies to certain foods.

Forms of Arthritis

There are two major forms of arthritic disease: rheumatoid arthritis and osteoarthritis.

Rheumatoid arthritis is a potentially crippling chronic disease that affects the joints of the entire skeleton rather than a single joint. It can be progressive—growing worse over time—but it is not always so. The disease occurs in women three times more often than men, and is most common in women between the ages of twenty and sixty. It generally appears between thirty-six and fifty. A juvenile form (juvenile rheumatoid arthritis) afflicts mostly females under age sixteen. It can begin as early as the age of six weeks, although it is more likely after six months. As in the adult form, infection and auto-immune deficiencies are suspected as causes, although research is incomplete and inconclusive.

Bones are attached to each other at joints. Joints that are designed to move are covered by slippery membranes and surrounded by sacs containing a lubricating fluid. The pain, swelling, inflammation, and stiffness of arthritis are the result of the destruction of the joint tissues and sometimes of the bone surface itself. The body attempts to repair the damage by producing scar tissue, but this merely closes up the spaces between the joints. At times the joints may actually fuse together.

81

Fatigue, weakness, anemia, weight loss due to poor appetite, and a low-grade fever are also symptoms of rheumatoid arthritis. The symptoms may disappear and recur again and again.

The most common form of arthritis, osteoarthritis, is a degenerative disease that is usually found in older people. It is the result of years of wear and tear on weight-bearing joints, most often the knees and hips. After many years of use or as the result of injury, the protective covering of cartilage over bone ends and joints wears thin. Eventually it may wear through and permit the rough surfaces of the bones to rub together. When that happens, the joint becomes painful and stiff. These symptoms may be especially troublesome in the morning, in cold, damp weather, or following strenuous activity. If the disease progresses, the joint may become inflamed.

Treatment
Although the exact causes of arthritis are unknown, some researchers believe there is a nutritional factor. It is known, for example, that rheumatoid arthritis sufferers have high levels of copper and low levels of iron in their blood. They also have high levels of iron in their joints and lymph glands and this may be the cause of joint pain. Some think poor nutrition itself may be a cause of arthritis.

The possible link between arthritis and diet has been debated for many years and many nutritional cures have been claimed. Research on the nutritional link is ongoing. Recently, for example, fish oils that contain certain fatty acids have been thought to reduce the symptoms of some forms of arthritis. The fatty acids are said to reduce joint inflammation.[2]

Some physicians and patients believe the pain associated with arthritis is made worse by certain foods, such as red meat, pork, wheat, and dairy products.

They think that eliminating these items from the diet improves the condition. On the other hand, opponents suggest that these changes merely have a placebo effect—they reduce symptoms because the patient believes they will help. Doctors warn patients that it may be dangerous to eliminate important food groups from the diet, particularly for older people whose nutrition may already be inadequate.

Because so many people are afflicted with the disease, and because it produces chronic pain, many sufferers fall prey to so-called "cures" that do no good and may be harmful because the victim may neglect the proper treatment for the condition.

The basic treatment for arthritis is still rest, proper exercise, anti-inflammatory medication, and taking off excess pounds if overweight. A well-balanced diet is also recommended so the body can get all the nutrients it needs to repair damage and fight infection and inflammation.

BEHAVIORAL DISORDERS

The idea that food affects behavior has been around for a very long time. Primitive societies thought plants and animals had powers that could be transferred to whoever ate them. Someone who ate a lion's heart would gain the lion's courage, for example, or the timidity attributed to a weak creature or plant would pass to anyone who made a meal of it. Perhaps the best-known example of the belief that food affects behavior is the biblical story of Adam and the apple.

The idea that food and behavior are linked is still common. An advertising slogan suggesting a certain food product contains "nature's goodness" is similar to the belief that a lion's heart contains "courage." However, scientific studies have shown links between some foods and behavior. A lack of vitamin B_1, for example, is thought to produce irritability, anger, and aggressiveness—characteristics that are associated with antisocial behavior. Some researchers therefore suggest that a deficiency of B vitamins in the diet may be associated with delinquency and criminal behavior. As another example, the Feingold Association (supporters of a pediatric allergist who developed the theory) maintains that certain foods, food colors, and food additives can cause hyperactivity and other unwanted behaviors in susceptible children. The American Medical Association has not accepted this thesis.

Any claim that directly links food with specific behavior is questionable. Because social, cultural, and personal attitudes are important, the strength of one's belief about what a food can do is likely to be greater than what can be documented. Unless other possible causes of observed behavior are ruled out, reports that claim behavior is food-linked may be inaccurate, especially since the effects of nutrients on the brain are still largely unknown. Also, the findings from animal studies of the effects of food on behavior may not always apply to people. Further, anxiety, depression, irritability, hyperactivity, fatigue, insomnia, and other types of behavior can have causes unrelated to diet.

Although it is not a food or a nutrient, caffeine is common in the American diet. About three-fourths of all caffeine consumed in the United States is in coffee, but it is also found in tea and is added to many cola drinks.

In small amounts, caffeine is a mild central nervous system stimulant. Large doses can affect behavior. In addition, some research suggests that excessive coffee drinking (six cups or more a day) may increase the cholesterol level. This has been contradicted by other studies. This controversy is an example of the uncertainty of the links between diet and disease.

Generally it is believed that moderate doses of caffeine may improve performance and feelings of alertness, but the degree varies with the individual. Children who are unused to caffeine may become anxious, while people whose tolerance for caffeine is high may have no adverse effects. Withdrawal from caffeine can produce a variety of symptoms including headache, lethargy, and irritability.

Eating Disorders

Obesity, anorexia nervosa, bulimia, and pica are diet-related conditions that influence what and how much people eat.

Obesity, or excessive body fat, results when more calories are consumed than are burned. The causes of over-eating include learned behavior and genetic influences—obesity frequently is a family problem—as well as impaired food intake regulating mechanisms.

The eating patterns of obese people are abnormal; their personalities may change and, as a result, they may make behavioral changes to accommodate their obesity. See page 99 for more on obesity.

A dramatic behavioral change—self-starvation—characterizes anorexia nervosa. Teenage girls, often "model children," are usually affected, although it is sometimes seen in older women. It is ten times more common among females than males, perhaps affecting 5 percent of females in North America.[3] The time of greatest risk is around the onset of puberty, when looks and body image take on undue importance. The disorder may begin following a death, parental divorce, broken romance, sexual encounter, or other stressful event, although minor events may also be precipitating factors.

The causes of anorexia nervosa are not known but may include physiological, psychological, family, and social problems. Victims are reluctant to undergo treatment because gaining weight is precisely what the anorectic is trying to avoid.

Anorexia nervosa is very serious and may lead to death in 15 to 21 percent of those with the condition. Hospitalization is often required to prevent death from starvation. Psychiatric disorders and the cessation of monthly periods in girls are signs of this diet-related disorder.

Undereating that is not anorexic behavior but is intended to lose weight or maintain a weight level can also be hazardous. It may produce chronic fatigue that makes exercise, an important component of dieting, difficult. Also, because the body's metabolism is slowed when undereating, resuming a normal diet may produce a weight gain.[4]

Approximately 50 percent of anorectics and a smaller percentage of obese people practice a cycle of excessive over-eating (binging) followed by purging the food from the body by vomiting or by using laxatives. This eating disorder, bulimia, is most common in teenage to early thirties females. Its onset may begin with a real or perceived need to lose weight through dieting, which then becomes a preoccupation.[5]

Researchers' reports vary widely and state that from 20 to 80 percent of American high school and college women occasionally practice bingeing/purging. Estimates are that about 8 percent practice it regularly. Binge eating usually involves foods that are "forbidden." The guilt of overeating is then reduced or eliminated by getting rid of the food. The cycle may be repeated over and over.

Serious medical problems such as torn stomach and esophageal linings, dehydration, kidney problems, urinary infections, tooth decay, and even heart attack may result from this disorder.

Pica is a disorder in which nonfood substances such as clay, starch, paint chips, chalk, paste, wax, hair, earth, and other things are intentionally and compulsively eaten. Although it is an eating disorder, it is not necessarily caused by poor nutrition. The specific causes are not known although some researchers suspect that craving and eating nonfood material may be a way to handle stress, get calcium, iron, and other nutrients into the diet, or prevent the nausea that sometimes accompanies pregnancy. These theories are unproven.

Effects of Food Colors and Additives
Numerous substances are added to food to enhance its appearance, prolong its shelf life, and generally make it more appealing and easier to sell. There are hundreds of additives used in commercial foods today, and their effects on people are not fully understood.

A hundred years ago food manufacturers secretly added chemicals to their products to preserve them or improve their color. Formaldehyde, the chemical used in embalming, was added to milk to keep it from spoiling. Copper was added to canned peas to brighten their color. Flour was mixed into expensive spices to increase their bulk and weight. At that time, most consumers bought much of their food fresh, from people they knew, and the effects of the abuse were limited.

The practice of adulterating food products spread as mass production and marketing methods were devised to get food to a growing population. The need to ship foods over long distances made spoilage a serious problem for producers, processors, and food retailers. New additives were invented and innovations such as putting plaster of Paris in candy and adding sawdust to black pepper and bread were used to prevent economic loss. Such practices were often followed without regard for their potential danger.

People began to be concerned about food safety by the turn of the century. In the early 1900s, a pure-food activist, Dr. Harvey Wiley, crusaded for food industry regulation, particularly for the removal of sodium nitrate as a preservative for sausage and bacon. This chemical is still used, however, even though it is known that nitrates and nitrites form nitrosamines, which are considered carcinogenic (cancer-producing).

At about the same time, public indignation was aroused by novelist Upton Sinclair's powerful book, *The Jungle*, which described the filthy conditions in the Chicago meat-packing industry. A single line from the book shows why. Describing how thousands of rats infested meat storage rooms, Sinclair wrote, "These rats were nuisances, and the packers would put poisoned bread out for them; they would die, and then rats, bread, and meat would go into the hoppers together." To make sausage!

An undercover federal investigation ordered by President Theodore Roosevelt discovered that the conditions in the meat-packing industry were even worse than those Sinclair described. As a result, the Pure Food Law was adopted in 1907. Although improper food processing and packaging practices continued, often masked by imaginative labeling and advertising, some abuses were stopped.

Then hundreds of new additives were developed, so that by the end of the Second World War in 1945, the Food and Drug Administration (enforcing the Food, Drug and Cosmetic Act of 1938) could not keep up with them, and many were not tested. In the 1960s, consumption of processed and convenience food soared. Estimates suggest that the average American eats two to three pounds of chemical additives annually. The full effects of these substances in the diet is still not known.

The Feingold Association (see p. 84) and other groups claim food additives may produce hyperactivity—inattention, excessive movement, impulsive behavior, learning disabilities, and inappropriate conduct—in children. However, statistical analyses of the results of studies investigating the effects of food additives on children have not provided evidence to support this belief. The studies included investigations of artificial food dyes, sugar, and caffeine. Even so, some medical authorities believe the suggestion that diet may contribute to behavior disorders in children must be taken seriously.

CANCER

Cancer, the uncontrolled growth of body cells, is second only to heart disease as a leading cause of death in the United States. For two thousand years people have suspected that cancer and diet were linked.

Twentieth-century research led scientists to believe that certain foods—including whole grain bread, milk, and cabbage and related vegetables—provided some protection against cancer and that people who were overweight ran a higher risk of developing cancer than those who were underweight. Animal studies showed that certain cancers were more likely in rats fed high-fat diets and that when underfed, rats had lower incidences of the disease. However, little effort was made to connect the findings with human cancer.

Cancer has been linked to certain nutrients, but the connections are not fully understood. Some protein-rich foods, charcoal-broiled meats and fish, and pickled, cured, salted, and smoked foods have been associated with cancer, but most research has been done with animals, and the findings may not apply to human beings.[6]

In the 1960s, interest in the link between nutrition and human cancer was revived when the World Health Organization issued a report on possible connections between cancer and life-style and environmental factors, and concluded that most human cancer may be preventable. New research focused on the link, and the result has been a wealth of scientific data that associates diet with the disease. An estimated 40 percent of cancer deaths in men and 60 percent of cancer deaths in women (some researchers say 50 percent for both men and women) is nutrition-linked and may be preventable by changes in the diet. Those changes should begin early in life. For example, the risk of colon cancer is believed to be increased for children whose diets are rich in processed luncheon meats and fried foods.[7] On the other hand, childhood diets rich in peanut butter, low-fat milk and cheese, nonfried foods and cabbage-related vegetables apparently have an anticarcinogenic effect.

Dietary Fat and Cancer

Fat is an important nutrient that has a direct effect on many cell functions. Consistent evidence from numerous animal and human studies suggests a connection between dietary fat and cancers of the breast,[8] colon, rectum, ovaries, endometrium (the mucous membrane lining the uterus), and prostate gland. Dietary fat may cause cancer directly by damaging the lining of the colon, for example, or indirectly by producing chemical or hormonal changes that in turn support cancer in various tissues. The National Research Council suggests reducing the consumption of fat to lower the risk of cancer of the colon, prostate, and breast.[9] It recommends limiting fats to 30 percent of total daily calorie consumption by avoiding fatty meats and whole-milk dairy products. Currently, the average American gets 37 percent of his or her calories from fat. Switching to fish, lean meats, skinless poultry, and low-fat dairy products is suggested. Studies on rats at Cornell University suggest that adding fish oil to the diet may reduce the risk of pancreatic cancer.

Calories and Cancer

Studies show that calorie intake and cancer are connected, although the full significance of the link is not yet understood.

Over-nutrition in animals has been shown to increase the risk of cancer, although there is no explanation of why this happens. Experiments also suggest that laboratory animals whose lifelong caloric intake has been restricted have less cancer, and that there is less cancer even in those who have had their calories limited as adults.

A large population study by the American Cancer Society reported cancer mortality to be lowest in people whose body weights were slightly under to slightly over averages based on age and height. Other studies state that men and women who are more than 40 percent heavier than average have a 33 percent (for men) and a 55 percent (for women) higher death rate from cancer.

Dietary Fiber and Cancer

Dietary fiber is a component of plants known to be important to human nutrition, although its effects on digestion are not fully understood. Some fibers speed the passage of food material through the alimentary canal, some affect the absorption of nutrients from food and, in general, fiber is believed to influence the growth of intestinal bacteria. The principal types of dietary fiber are either soluble or insoluble. Soluble fiber, which is found in many fruits and some grains, is broken down by bacterial action in the colon into fatty acids that are absorbed into the body.[10] Insoluble fiber, which is found in whole grains, wheat bran, corn, and lentils, is not broken down. A balance of both kinds of fibers in the diet is recommended for good health.

The major sources of dietary fiber are fruits, vegetables, and whole-grain cereals. For most of history, normal diets contained large amounts of these foods,

91

so there was ample fiber in the average diet. In the United States and many developed nations, increased consumption of refined foods from which much or all of the fiber has been removed has led to a number of problems. It is estimated that the average intake of dietary fiber in these countries has been reduced to 20 percent of what it was only a century ago. Gastrointestinal upsets, diverticulitis (the inflammation of the lower intestinal wall), constipation, and diseases of the digestive system have become common. The increase of cancer of the colon also has been linked in human and animal studies to the reduction of dietary fiber.

Why fiber seems to protect against cancer and other diseases is still under investigation, but contributing factors may include a shorter time that wastes are held in the colon, reduced production of potential carcinogens, and the dilution of carcinogens already present in the colon. Some researchers believe it is not the fiber itself that is beneficial but the replacement of fats in the diet with grain. Nutritionists suggest Americans' health would benefit if daily dietary fiber were doubled. The National Cancer Institute recommends a daily fiber intake of 20 to 30 grams.[11] The idea is to replace high-fat foods with foods high in fiber, not to supplement them. People who are not used to high-fiber diets who increase their daily fiber consumption should begin slowly and drink six to eight glasses of water daily until their systems adjust.

CORONARY HEART DISEASE

Coronary heart disease, a general term for cardiac disorders caused by poor blood circulation to the heart muscle, begins quietly, perhaps as early as between ten and fifteen years of age, or even in infancy. It is usually the result of atherosclerosis (narrowed arteries due to fatty deposits called plaque) that may be precipitated by high blood cholesterol, high blood pressure, and cigarette smoking—all of which are under a person's control to change. Each year, more people die of coronary heart disease—mostly heart attacks—than any other disease, though fortunately, the death rate is declining. Excessive cholesterol is sometimes the diet-linked factor in this disease.

Cholesterol

Shortly after the start of the twentieth century, researchers produced atherosclerosis in animals by feeding them diets rich in fat and cholesterol. (Earlier investigations already had identified blood cholesterol and plaque.) In other studies, observations of the dietary patterns of various human populations seemed to confirm a connection between coronary heart disease and certain kinds of foods. People whose diets were high in vegetables had little coronary heart disease, while groups who ate lots of animal products such as meat, butter, and eggs, had much higher rates of the disease. It is now known that diets high in animal fat contain high levels of cholesterol, and that high levels of blood cholesterol are linked to coronary heart disease.

Not all researchers agree that cholesterol is the culprit in producing heart disease.[12] On the other hand, some new research suggests that the connection may be even greater than previously thought. This controversy is one example from among the many possible that demonstrates how difficult it is for people to know what is and is not good for their health. In this controversy, there is a consensus in the medical community that a low-fat, low-cholesterol diet is recommended for everyone except children under two. The guidelines suggest limiting calories from fat to 30 percent of total caloric intake, limiting saturated fat to

93

less than 10 percent, and limiting cholesterol to less than 300 mg daily. It is believed that if these recommendations were followed, the incidence of coronary heart disease among Americans could be reduced by about 20 percent. Other factors linked to heart disease include smoking, obesity, high blood pressure, and a family history of the disease.

Other Dietary Links

Obesity, alcohol consumption, carbohydrate intake, coffee drinking, and other dietary factors have been investigated with the objective of determining their roles in coronary heart disease.

Obesity has been directly linked with an increased risk of heart disease, and evidence suggests that losing weight reduces the risk. People who are overweight in the upper-abdominal area run a greater risk of coronary heart disease, high blood pressure, stroke, and diabetes than those who gain weight in the lower body. This may account for the fact that overweight women who tend to carry excess fat in the hips and thighs are generally healthier than overweight men whose fat is stored in the abdomen.[13]

Studies of alcohol use have produced conflicting results. For example, one study concluded that two drinks a day increase a woman's risk of developing breast cancer by 50 percent. Another found that moderate alcohol consumption reduces a woman's chances of developing heart disease by 40 to 60 percent. Studies that suggest that moderate alcohol consumption reduces the risk of coronary heart disease by increasing levels of beneficial cholesterol (cholesterol manufactured by the liver and essential for well-being) are offset by other, recent investigations that contradict this conclusion by suggesting that alcohol does not increase the blood levels of so-called "good" cholesterol. Because other negative effects of alcohol far outweigh its questionable benefits in coronary heart disease, its use is not recommended.

Diets high in unrefined or minimally processed carbohydrates are usually high in dietary fiber and low in fat. People who follow such diets may be lowering the risk of coronary heart disease.

There is no agreement on the effects of sugar on coronary heart disease. Some researchers claim a link while others refute it. Similarly, no strong evidence has been found of a link between vitamin and mineral intake and high cholesterol levels or coronary heart disease.

DIABETES

Although people have known about the disease diabetes for 2,500 years, and a nutrition link has also long been known, there always has been disagreement among physicians and researchers about the best way to treat the disease. Even today, except for the general approach of limiting calories and encouraging weight reduction, no single dietary therapy has proved to be better than another in treating people with adult-onset diabetes.

About 11 million Americans suffer from diabetes, a chronic disease characterized by improper metabolism of carbohydrate, fat, and protein. Only about 5 million are diagnosed. The rest do not know they are diabetic. Diabetes is caused by the production of too little of the hormone insulin, or by the resistance of the body's cells to the action of the hormone. Diabetes is the seventh major cause of death in the United States, leading directly to 36,000 deaths annually. Almost 100,000 additional deaths are due to complications associated with diabetes, particularly cardiovascular disease and strokes. Diabetes also causes most new blindness (acquired adult blindness), about 5,000 cases a year in people between ages twenty and seventy-four.

There is no cure for diabetes, but effective treatment to control it permits those who have the disease to live near-normal to completely normal lives. There are two major forms of diabetes: Type I, insulin dependent diabetes mellitus, formerly called juvenile-onset diabetes; and Type II, noninsulin dependent diabetes mellitus, formerly called adult-onset diabetes. Type II is by far the more common, accounting for about 90 percent of all diabetes.

Type I diabetes begins suddenly, usually affecting young people around the age of ten or twelve, although it may appear as late as forty, and is caused by a major deficiency of the hormone insulin. Treatment includes the administration of insulin as well as strict control of the diet. Approximately 1 million Americans suffer from this form of the disease.

The vastly more common form of diabetes, Type II, usually begins around middle age, most often in overweight or obese people. It begins gradually and may not produce visible symptoms. The cause is often a resistance of the body cells to the action of the body's insulin rather than an actual lack of the hormone. Treatment relies heavily on carefully controlling the diet to keep weight down. An estimated 10 to 12 million Americans have Type II diabetes, although most do not know it.

Dietary treatment of diabetes has been prescribed for centuries. Early Egyptians suffering from the disease, with symptoms of wasting away and frequent urination, were given a diet of wheat, grapes, honey, and berries. A diet of milk, cereals, fruits, and sweet wine was prescribed in Roman times. A seventeenth-century diet called for milk, bread, and barley water. The common nutrient in these diets was carbohydrate.

Later diets avoided carbohydrates and called instead for foods high in protein. One—hardly tempting even to save a life—consisted of blood pudding made with suet and rancid meat. When it was noticed that the amount of sugar passed in the urine—a symptom of diabetes—fell when food was scarce, semistarvation was prescribed. Other treatments restricted carbohydrates and protein, and total caloric intake as well. All treatments were affecting blood sugar levels, although the exact biochemical mechanism was unknown. Currently, the American Heart Association and the American Diabetes Association recommend a diet consisting of 50 to 60 percent carbohydrates. Some researchers disagree, however, because they believe people with insulin resistance may run a higher risk of heart disease on a high-carbohydrate diet. Instead, they recommend a diet of 40 to 45 percent carbohydrates for insulin-resistant people.[14]

Research has shown that diabetes does not occur in hunter-gatherer populations with a high-fiber natural diet.[15] Gallstones, colon cancer, diverticulitis, and heart attacks are also rare or nonexistent in these cultures.

In 1921 researchers extracted insulin from the pancreatic tissue of dogs. Insulin is a hormone produced in specialized cells of the pancreas; it regulates blood sugar levels. Because high blood sugar is a major characteristic of diabetes, insulin plays an important role in controlling the disease by lowering it. Once this aspect of diabetes was understood, treatment for diabetes was more certain, but strict control of diet continues to be essential. Researchers have also found evidence that vitamin C is an important component in diabetes treatment, and have suggested that supplements of this vitamin may help patients' resistance to some of the side effects of diabetes, notably blindess, kidney damage, slow wound healing, and gangrene.[16]

HIGH BLOOD PRESSURE

A dramatic example of how using a recognized link between nutrition and disease can lead to treatments yielding health benefits is that of high blood pressure, or hypertension.

Cardiovascular disease, the term for a number of abnormal conditions of the circulatory system, ranks as the primary cause of death in the United States, accounting for 50 percent of all deaths from disease annually. High blood pressure is a significant contributor to cardiovascular disease. Approximately 15 to 20 percent of adult Americans are hypertensive. According to one researcher who studied the correlation between high levels of cholesterol and hypertension, a large percentage of American children will develop hypertension as adults because the cholesterol levels of about one-fourth to one-third of them are close to the danger level (over 176 milligrams per 100 milliters of blood).

In the past twenty years, public awareness of the dangers of high blood pressure and the subsequent efforts to detect and treat this condition have doubled the number of people who have brought their blood pressure under control. Early detection is essential because hypertension generally does not produce symptoms until it has actually damaged the heart, vascular system, brain, or kidneys.

The death rate from cardiovascular disease dropped over 42 percent in the period from the mid-1960s to the mid-1980s. Although a large percentage of this decrease is attributed to the reduction of cholestrol in the blood, treatment for high blood pressure and other changes in life-style have also contributed to this improving health picture.

Blood pressure is a measure of the internal pressure of the cardiovascular system. Two readings are taken when blood pressure is measured. The systolic pressure is the pressure against the walls of the arteries, veins, and heart, when the heart contracts to pump blood. The pulse of blood rushing through the system increases the pressure just as a burst of water does as it surges through a garden hose when the faucet is opened. The second measurement, the diastolic pressure, is the pressure on the circulating system when the heart is relaxed.

Normal blood pressure for a healthy, twenty-one-year-old male is commonly written as 120/80 (read as 120 over 80) and 110/70 for a similar female. Normal blood pressure for children ages ten to nineteen is 105/65. The first reading is an indication of how hard the heart works to pump blood through the system. The second reading is the constant pressure on the system. The higher the numbers, the harder the heart is working.

Blood pressure varies with age, weight, diet, and other factors. Regular exercise, for example, can significantly reduce blood pressure. Long distance runners typically have low blood pressure readings which are an indication of the sound health of their hearts.

Overweight has a major effect on raising blood pressure. Diet, particularly the consumption of sodium—mostly in salt—also contributes significantly. Treatment for high blood pressure almost always includes the requirement to lose weight and to reduce the amount of salt in the diet.

OBESITY

No condition that affects health is so clearly related to diet as is obesity, or excessive body fat. It is also one of the most common conditions, with over 30 million American adults between the ages of twenty and seventy-four abnormally overweight. Studies suggest that obesity and extreme obesity in children and teenagers is increasing dramatically. The rise in the number of obese children, ages six through eleven, for example, has been more than 50 percent since the mid-1960s.

Research indicates that genetics plays a significant role. Children of obese parents are three to four times more likely to be overweight than children of lean parents. Also, studies show that approximately one-fourth of an individual's excess fat is genetically linked; environmental influences account for the rest.

Obesity is generally defined as a body weight 20 percent above normal as designated in height–weight charts. Basically, obesity is the result of high calorie intake and inadequate energy expenditure due to biochemical, hormonal, genetic, psychological, and other factors. Ideal ranges of body fat are 12 to 15 percent of body weight for men and 22 to 25 percent for women.[17]

Although obesity alone does not automatically mean poor health, the condition increases the risk for high blood cholesterol, hypertension, diabetes, coronary heart disease, kidney and gallbladder disease, and some cancers. Studies show that increased weight is linked to increased mortality. Its effect on mental health may also be significant.

Obesity is probably a modern condition, created partly by the ease with which food became available. It was unknown in England, for example, until the 1700s. The industrial revolution and subsequent advances in agricultural production, transportation of foodstuffs to the marketplace, and food processing all made it easy to obtain food.

Moderate obesity has been used as a symbol of health, fertility, and beauty at various times in history. Rubens's full-figured women are an example. On the other hand, a medical condition called Pickwickian syndrome—named for Charles Dickens's extremely obese Mr. Pickwick—demonstrates the realization that there is a connection between obesity and poor health.

If simple overeating were the cause of obesity, the cure—dieting—would be obvious. Eating less while exercising more are steps to reduce obesity. However, because there are genetic, hormonal, metabolic, behavioral, and psychological components to obesity, the answer is not so simple. About 65 million Americans go on diets each year, although most of these people are not obese but merely overweight. Unfortunately, an estimated 90 percent of those who diet to lose weight gain it back. Obesity—extreme overweight—may be symptomatic of other problems which also need treatment.

SKELETAL DISEASES

An interesting change has occurred in the relationship of diet to diseases that affect the bones. In the past, rickets, a vitamin D deficiency disease, was common among children, particularly after the Industrial Revolution and the dramatic social and economic changes it created. Crowded, substandard living conditions, poor nutrition, and limited exposure to sunshine created the perfect conditions for the spread of a disease that had been known since early times, but had been relatively rare.

Until very recently, very few people lived to old age. Now, as the upper limits of longevity are being challenged, a new diet-related bone disease, osteoporosis, has become a serious concern. Rickets, the disease that affects children, has been virtually eradicated in developed nations, while in those same countries, whose population increasingly enjoys longer lives, osteoporosis has become prevalent.

Rickets

Rickets is a disease of infancy and childhood that is characterized by abnormal bone formation, soft, pliable bones, and a number of skeletal abnormalities including bowlegs, knock-knees, and a curved spine. It is the result of a diet deficient in vitamin D, calcium, and often, phosphorus.

The disease was mostly associated with children living in crowded, substandard conditions common in cities. As recently as 1921, three-fourths of all children in New York City may have suffered from rickets.

Although cod liver oil, which is rich in vitamin D, was used to treat rickets in the early 1800s, it was not until the twentieth century that diet, sunshine, and living conditions were recognized as factors in the disease. Rickets is uncommon today in the United States, in large measure because of the addition of vitamin D to milk and improved diets and health conditions.

Osteoporosis

Bone tissue is made mainly of protein, calcium, and phosphorus. Healthy bone is about as strong as a piece of hickory wood of the same size. However bone, like most body tissues, is in a continuous cycle of formation, breakdown, and re-formation. Until young adulthood, bone formation dominates the cycle, and bones grow stronger. But by about age thirty-five and beyond, bone begins to break down more than it builds, and bones lose strength. Because men have greater bone mass than women, women's bones are generally weaker.

The loss of bone mass is called osteoporosis. The result of this disease is weak bones that are easily broken. When a young person breaks a bone, it is able to heal faster and more efficiently than a similar break in someone older. Also, hormonal changes in women after menopause increase bone loss so that women, as

102

a group, suffer more from the effects of osteoporosis, though males also lose bone mass.

A serious complication of osteoporosis in older people is that a serious bone break, most commonly in the hip, may lead to a downward health spiral. An elderly person's health, which already may be marginal, may plummet when slow-healing, calcium-poor bones keep them bedridden and later limit their activity.

Although osteoporosis is generally associated with older people, it is a serious concern for the young because the condition begins in youth. It is estimated that an average adolescent girl today gets little more than half the calcium in her diet that she needs. Because bone-building is at its peak in young women, a reduced calcium diet will produce weaker, less dense bones. When the girl grows older, bone mass deterioration will be significantly greater because the bones were less dense to begin with. Today's high consumption of processed foods and soft drinks made with phosphorus contributes to the problem since elevated phosphorus levels in the body increase calcium loss.

Increased calcium intake is not the whole solution to the prevention of osteoporosis, however. Prevention begins in youth with the start of a lifelong program of a healthy, calcium-rich diet, no smoking, and regular exercise to promote maximum bone growth and strength.

GASTROINTESTINAL DISEASES

It's not surprising that the digestive system is the starting point of many nutrition-related diseases since it is in this system that food is converted into usable form. Improper digestion and absorption lead to malnutrition, the improper nourishment of body cells, and disease. For example, if iron is not present or cannot be absorbed from digested food, anemia may result. Too much fat in the diet may lead to obesity as well as a host of other diseases. The digestive system is also subject to nutrition-related diseases. These include cancer, liver disease, gallbladder disease and ulcers, as well as less serious but still distressing conditions such as diverticulitis, appendicitis, and constipation. Each has specific—although not always known—causes. Liver disease (cirrhosis) is linked with excessive alcohol use. Ulcers are associated with excessive acid production which has been suggested, although not proved, to be promoted by highly refined foods.

A common factor in a number of gastrointestinal diseases is dietary fiber, the undigestible portion of plants. Dietary fiber is made of a number of different materials, and each can have an effect on the digestive system. Some affect the ability of the colon to hold water, others speed the passage of digested food, and some affect the production of beneficial bacteria.

Diverticular disease is an example of how fiber affects the gastrointestinal system. Diverticulosis is a condition that is found more often in industrialized Western nations and least often in developing nations. Differences in diet are thought to be a principal cause. People in industrialized nations such as the United States tend to have diets that are high in refined foods. Food in less developed countries is often less refined. Since it is known that refining food removes much of the natural fiber, the conclusion is that a lack of fiber in the diet leads to diverticular disease. Studies support this conclusion.

The walls of the intestine are lined with mucous tissue. Behind this is muscle tissue. When pressure in the large intestine gets too high, the inner mucous-tissue lining forms bulges in the muscle tissue. These bulges or sacs (diverticula) may fill with solid matter passing through the intestine. Diverticulitis, an inflammation of these sacs, occurs if they become infected.

Diets high in fiber minimize this and similar gastrointestinal diseases by providing bulk, increasing water retention, and speeding the passage of solid wastes through the intestine. Dietary fiber supplements are often used to treat diverticular disease.

OTHER NUTRITION-DISEASE LINKS

The connection between diet and disease is not limited to a few, well-known diseases and medical conditions. Nutrition is fundamental to good health and every aspect of health is affected by it. General good health is each person's defense system against relatively benign conditions like simple infections as well as serious, life-threatening diseases.

Infection

Connections between malnutrition and infection have been suspected for centuries. Plagues, outbreaks of dysentery, typhus and smallpox, epidemics of typhoid, measles, and other diseases were often seen during famines and wars—times when food was scarce, inadequate, or contaminated.

Through the centuries, efforts to improve sanitation, purify public water supplies, and assure production and delivery of pure food, along with programs of immunization against specific diseases, have reduced or eliminated many infectious diseases. Although the virtual eradication of such infectious diseases as measles, mumps, and rubella is the result of vaccines, nutritional status is a significant factor too: It is known to affect the body's immune response to these and other diseases, and good nutrition is an essential component in their control.

Immunity

Malnutrition is known to have a negative effect on the body's immune system although it is not fully understood.[18] When severely malnourished, the body is unable to fight disease with its usual arsenal of weapons, which includes fever and the increased production of white cells. A body weakened by malnutrition is also more susceptible to diseases that a healthy body would withstand. The effects of nutrition on the immune system are just beginning to be investigated. Special diets have been shown to reduce infection rates among burn patients, protect against postoperative infections, and possibly retard the progress of AIDS-related infections.

AIDS is a dramatic example of the complex relationship among infection, nutrition, and immunity in a disease. The devastation and ultimate death seen in AIDS is caused by multiple, immune-related diseases and infections.

Although it is unproven if nutritional therapy can stop or reverse the progress of AIDS-related diseases, it is known that HIV-infected patients who are malnourished are at the greatest risk. Typically, the patient experiences anorexia, nausea, vomiting, fever, diarrhea, intestinal injury, and poor absorption of nutrients. Researchers believe that the malnutrition associated with AIDS is more likely a result of the disease than its cause.

Dental Disease

Nutrition-related dental disease is not limited to diseases like scurvy, with its dramatic symptoms of falling teeth and bleeding gums. Ordinary dental caries—"cavities"—are also linked to diet. Even the Greeks of ancient times knew that sweets produced tooth decay. It wasn't until the late 1800s that experiments showed how carbohydrates mixed with saliva to eat away the hard surface of teeth, exposing the softer inner part to decay.

Normally developed teeth have a durable mineral coating that resists decay as well as general wear and tear from chewing. This coating is built up as the tooth grows. It continues to gain strength after the tooth erupts from the gum, absorbing minerals such as fluoride from food and saliva. Improper nutrition during tooth development produces a thin coating that is readily worn away or easily broken down by decaying food matter. The gums are also weakened by improper nutrition and are subject to diseases such as gingivitis.

Infant Health
Nutrition plays an especially important role in health at two very critical times of life, the periods of fetal development and childhood. It is during these times that an individual's basic growth occurs and the health baseline for the rest of his or her life is set. If a mother, during pregnancy, has poor nutrition, her developing child will suffer. Similarly, a child who eats poorly also will not develop adequately. The weak foundation created by inadequate nutrition during the critical formative years is compounded until maximum growth is attained, generally in the late teens. The final result is an adult with built-in susceptibilities for poor health because one or more body systems or functions are weak or deficient.

Birth weight is a measure of an infant's nutritional status and growth. A low birth weight increases an infant's chances of illness and mortality while heavier babies are more likely to be healthy. Adequate nutrition during pregnancy increases birth weight, and even mothers who begin a pregnancy poorly nourished can improve their odds of having a healthy baby by eating well. Good nutrition during pregnancy also improves the mother's health.

PMS (Premenstrual Syndrome)

The uncomfortable effects of premenstrual syndrome, an assortment of physical and emotional symptoms affecting some women in the days preceding their menstrual periods, may be reduced by eating six small meals daily, instead of the usual three, reducing stress, and cutting down on sugar, sodium, and caffeine. Foods rich in vitamin B_6, magnesium, vitamin E, potassium, and zinc are suggested.[19]

Neurologic Disorders

The full effects of nutrition on overall health are still under investigation and much remains unknown. Knowledge of the effects of nutrition on the brain and central nervous system are equally incomplete. Studies of these effects are made more difficult by a "blood-brain barrier" which prevents or slows passage of materials from the blood to the central nervous system. In the case of harmful materials, the blood-brain barrier protects the central nervous system, but it also interferes with the study of the effects of nutrition on the brain as it cancels out the effects of fluctuations of nutrients in the blood. It can be assumed, however, that the brain and central nervous system need all the essential nutrients for healthy functioning.

Stroke, the third-ranking cause of death in the United States, occurs when a portion of the brain is deprived of its blood supply and brain cells die from lack of oxygen. The result is mild to severe neurological impairment, or death. Stroke is related to diet because the conditions that may lead to a stroke are often the result of circulatory diseases that are caused or made worse by poor nutrition. Diabetes, high blood pressure, atherosclerosis, and other circulatory system diseases increase the risk of stroke.

Headache is a less deadly but serious problem. Though headache has many causes, certain foods—chocolate, cheese, red wine, and monosodium glutamate, for example—have been suspected of bringing on the malady in some people.

Acne

The precise cause of acne, a mild to severe skin disease that affects millions of Americans, is unknown. Approximately 80 percent of all teenagers develop acne, although it may start later—at age twenty-five to thirty—especially among females.

Acne is commonly believed to be linked to diet, particularly those laden with "junk foods" such as chocolate, nuts, cola drinks, potato chips, french fries, and others high in fat. However, no scientific evidence supports this belief. Yet some people find that certain foods do trigger acne.

A number of factors influence the development of acne. Most important is heredity. If a parent had acne, his or her child is more likely to be affected. The condition usually begins at the onset of maturity, about age eleven for girls and age thirteen for boys. Boys tend to suffer more severe acne than girls as a result of increased activity of sebaceous (oil) glands in the skin stimulated by the production of male hormones. Certain drugs and medicines, exposure to oils and grease, stress, and strong emotions can also trigger or contribute to the development of acne.

While no scientific link has been demonstrated between acne and nutrition, avoidance of foods such as chocolate and potato chips, or drinks that may cause or aggravate acne is sensible.

109

Nutrition and Longevity

How long a person lives is dependent on many factors. Heredity is a major influence. One aspect of aging recently investigated suggests that reduced caloric intake—eating less—may extend life. Experiments with mice showed that underfed mice lived an average 50 percent longer than normally fed mice. The underfed mice received adequate amounts of essential nutrients, but were given 40 percent fewer calories.[20]

6 DIETARY ALTERNATIVES, FADS, AND FRAUDS

Food and nutrition have other, less tangible influences on life, aside from the need for nutrients for growth and health. There are important emotional, nonphysical, associations. A parent's encouragement to a child to "eat your vegetables" or a host's invitation to "have a second helping" reflect an aspect of food that goes beyond simple nutrition. In these and similar instances, food stands for a part of the relationship between people. For a parent and child, food often stands for love and security. For a host and guests, a fine dinner has similar, non-nutritive aims such as hospitality, acceptance, and friendship.

The power of food extends to other areas that have nothing to do with growing, healthy bodies or fighting disease. For some, food is also "magic." That is, many believe that food has special properties. A modern counterpart of the idea that "courage" resides in a lion's heart is the belief that bee pollen confers longevity.

Although science has debunked many early beliefs about the power of certain foods, the willingness to believe still hangs on. In the past, it was thought that potions, elixirs, and witch's brews could produce supernatural effects. Fed by superstition and some empirical evidence, such as the ability of certain foods

111

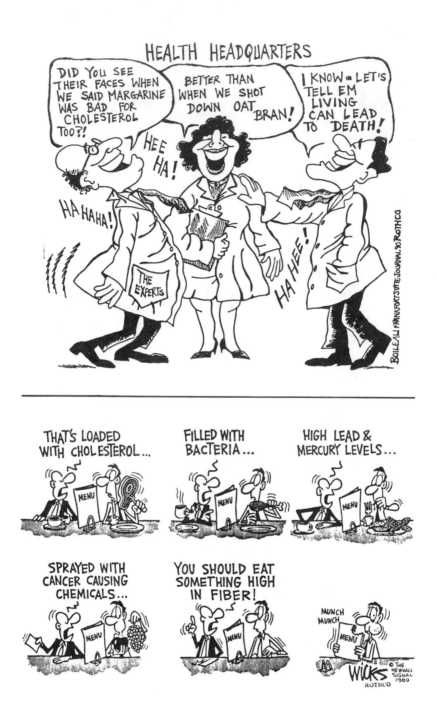

to produce hallucinations, deep sleep, or even death, the power of food was accepted by those whose wish was to believe. The strength of this acceptance is partly due to people's regional and cultural beliefs. These beliefs die hard because they are protected by a circle of believers and are shielded from outside information, questions, and conflicting opinions.

Sorcerers and scientists are thought to be privy to information that is unavailable or unknown to most people. When a person who wants to believe in magic is shown "magic" by someone claiming to know magic, the result is often an unquestioning acceptance of magic. Perhaps because food has strong emotional connotations, people tend to cling to their beliefs about its powers with unusual force. Proponents of the cancer-curing effects of a certain vitamin, for example, may remain unwilling to concede their belief was wrong even when evidence disproves the claim. Similarly, those who swear by "organically grown" foods will claim that "nonorganically grown" foods are unable to provide proper nutrition. Others will insist that only large doses of vitamins and other food supplements can assure good health.

A variety of beliefs about food and nutrition are held by many people. Some are flatly wrong, some are comprised of half-truths, and some are accurate to the best of anyone's ability to know. The result is often confusion and contradiction. And some of these beliefs result in out-and-out fraud.

Food faddism and fraud have had a long history in the United States. In 1630, a Massachusetts Bay Colony man was punished for selling an expensive but ineffective cure for scurvy. In the 1800s, the availability of newspapers and a large population that could read them created perfect conditions for advertising, and the potential for abusing it. "Snake oil" sellers roamed the country offering cures for everything from

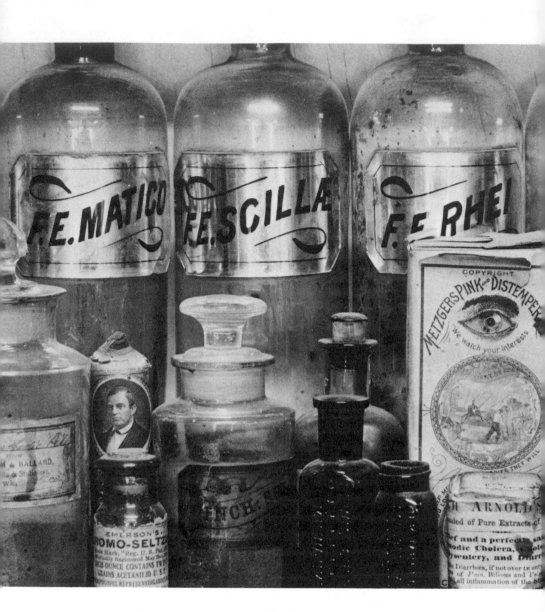

At various times in history, unproven
cures for everything from dandruff to
arthritis have appealed to people who wanted
to believe in the "cures'" healing powers.

dandruff to arthritis. Later, when nutritional discoveries such as vitamins were made, incomplete information was exploited to appeal to people's desires to believe in the curative power of food.

Today there are numerous conflicting claims made about food and its relationship to health. Some claims are based on simple avarice, the desire to make money from people's ignorance. Others are founded partly on fact and partly on fancy. Still others are based on conflicting studies by legitimate researchers. The result is often confusion, but more important, people's health may be compromised when nutritional decisions are made on the basis of misinformation or incomplete information. The danger is that when a myth or misinformation is believed, people may choose to follow the myth and defer medical advice or treatment. They may ingest untested, even toxic materials believing them to be health-giving. In addition, by clinging to an unproven belief, they don't allow themselves to learn about alternatives.

THE U.S. SURGEON GENERAL'S RECOMMENDATIONS

We've seen that health and diet are linked. We've also seen that the link often is incompletely known or understood, and that a lot of research remains to be done. In an attempt to consolidate what is currently known about diet and health into a comprehensive statement that people could use to make diet-related health decisions, the United States surgeon general commissioned a landmark report, *The Surgeon General's Report on Nutrition and Health*. The 1988 report makes a number of recommendations based on conclusions derived from scientific studies. The major issues the report addresses and the findings are:

115

Fats and cholesterol. Reduce consumption of fat, especially saturated fat, and cholesterol. Choose foods that are relatively low in these substances, such as vegetables, fruits, whole-grain foods, fish, poultry, lean meats, and low-fat dairy products. Use food preparation methods that add little or no fat.

Energy and weight control. Achieve and maintain a desirable body weight. To do so, choose a dietary pattern in which energy (caloric) intake is consistent with energy expenditure. To reduce energy intake, limit consumption of foods relatively high in calories, fats, and sugars and minimize alcohol consumption. Increase energy expenditure through regular and sustained physical exercise.

Complex carbohydrates and fiber. Increase consumption of whole-grain foods and cereal products, vegetables (including dried beans and peas), and fruits.

Sodium. Reduce intake of sodium by choosing foods relatively low in sodium and limiting the amount of salt added in food preparation and at the table.

Alcohol. To reduce the risk of chronic disease, take alcohol only in moderation (no more than two drinks a day), if at all. Avoid drinking any alcohol before or while driving, operating machinery, taking medications, or engaging in any activity requiring judgment. Avoid drinking alcohol while pregnant.

Fluoride. Community water systems should contain fluoride at optimal levels for prevention of tooth decay. If such water is not available, use other appropriate sources of fluoride.

Sugars. Those who are particularly vulnerable to dental caries (cavities), especially children, should limit their consumption of foods high in sugars.

Calcium. Adolescent girls and adult women should increase consumption of foods high in calcium, including low-fat dairy products.

Iron. Children, adolescents, and women of childbearing age should be sure to consume foods that are

116

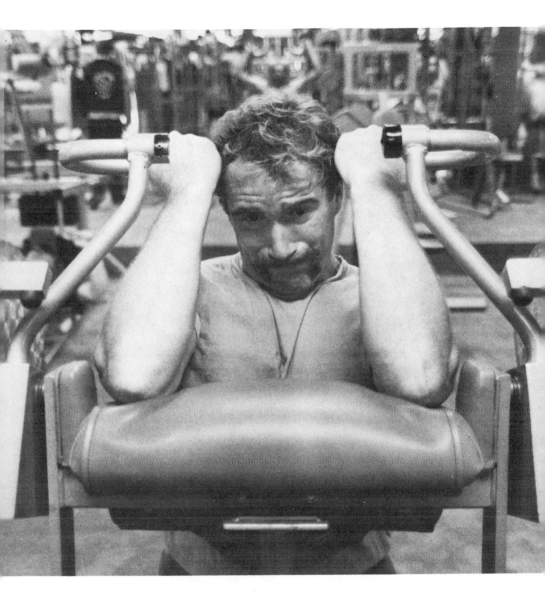

New research suggests that weight training is not just for athletes like football player Steve Shull. Along with a proper diet, it can be especially helpful for women in preventing osteoporosis.

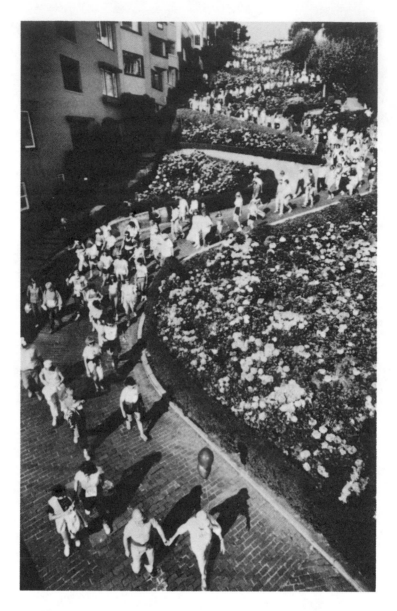

*This walkathon in San Francisco was organized
to promote walking as a fitness activity
in which anyone of any age can participate.*

good sources of iron, such as lean meats, fish, certain beans and iron-enriched cereals, and whole-grain products. This issue is of special concern for low-income families.

There is a growing body of evidence linking nutrition and disease. The early, unscientific observations of sailors and others whose health suffered because of poor diet have been replaced by massive studies and carefully controlled research. Now we have accumulating statistical proof to the adage, "You are what you eat." As it turns out, what and how we eat may be killing us. In the United States, for example, heart disease and cancer rates are among the highest in the world. Susceptibility to disease anywhere depends on much more than just diet, of course. Hereditary, environmental, and other factors contribute. But diet's role in the link between health and disease stands out sharply.

All of the answers to the connection between nutrition and disease have not been found. Some that are currently accepted may be disputed and changed. Controversy about what is good for you and what is not will continue to rise and fall as new information challenges old beliefs. In the meantime, being aware of what and how you eat, keeping informed of developments in health and nutrition, exercising moderation, and avoiding excess are simple ways to assure that the link between your nutrition and good health are strong.

SOURCE NOTES

INTRODUCTION
1. Rudolph Ballentine, M.D., *Diet & Nutrition,* (Honesdale, Pa.: Himalayan International Institute, 1978), 12–15.
2. *Ibid.* 157–159.

CHAPTER 1
1. Ruth L. Memmler and Dena L. Wood, *The Human Body in Health and Disease,* (Philadelphia: J.B. Lippincott, 1983), 332–334.

CHAPTER 2
1. B. T. Hunter, "Appreciating individual differences," *Consumers' Research Magazine,* November 1989, 8–9.

CHAPTER 3
1. "Kids' cholesterol," *Prevention,* March 1990, 20.
2. P. McCarthy, "Does protein build muscles?" *American Health,* November 1989, 96.
3. Rudolph Ballentine, M.D., *Diet and Nutrition,* (Honesdale, Pa.: Himalayan International Institute, 1978), 159.
4. J. Raloff, "Revised RDAs add a few good nutrients," *Science News,* October 28, 1989, 277.
5. T. Mendoza, "Mighty minerals in mini-doses," *Current Health,* December 1989, 22–25.
6. T. Mendoza, "The power of iron," *Current Health,* April 1989, 14–16.
7. A. Roblin, "New clues to the power of magnesium," *Prevention,* April 1989, 33–39.
8. R. A. Barnett, "Nuts about selenium," *American Health,* March 1989, 149.

CHAPTER 4
1. Rudolph Ballentine, M.D., *Diet & Nutrition*, (Honesdale, Pa.: Himalayan International Institute, 1978), 20.

CHAPTER 5
1. M. Beck, "Living with arthritis," *Newsweek*, March 20, 1989, 64–70.
2. G. L. Blackburn, "The anti-arthritis diet," *Prevention*, February 1989, 34–35.
3. D. Jenish, "A tragic obsession," *Maclean's*, October 9, 1989, 52.
4. F. Coleman, "The hazards of eating too little," *Women's Sports and Fitness*, March 1989, 18.
5. Patricia Long, *The Nutritional Ages of Women* (New York: Macmillan, 1986), 148–152.
6. T. Mendoza, "Diet, cancer, and common sense," *Current Health*, November 1989, 18–21.
7. "Reducing risk of colon cancer," *USA Today*, February 1989, 6.
8. J. Raloff, "Breast cancer rise: due to dietary fat?" *Science News*, April 21, 1990, 245.
9. "The diet-cancer link," *McCall's*, October 1989, 106.
10. M. Murray, "Confused about fiber?" *Reader's Digest*, July 1990, 75–78.
11. S. Stocker-Ferguson, "100 top fiber foods," *Prevention*, November 1989, 73.
12. J. Palca, "Getting to the heart of the cholesterol debate," *Science*, March 9, 1990, 1170–1171.
13. J. Poppy, "The paunch line," *Esquire*, February 1989, 59–60.
14. K. Fackelmann, "High carbohydrate diet may pose heart risks," *Science News*, September 16, 1989, 185.
15. "High fiber for diabetics," *The Saturday Evening Post*, January-February 1990, 12.
16. C. I. Nelson, "Diabetes and vitamin C," *New Choices for the Best Years*, May 1989, 15.
17. M. Bloom, "The fats of life," *World Tennis*, September 1989, 92–95.
18. C. Perlmutter, "Diet and immunity: the new frontier," *Prevention*, October 1989, 46–52.
19. "Oh, those menstrual blues," *Teen*, April 1990, 20.
20. "Curtailing calories may lengthen life," *FDA Consumer*, February 1989, 3–4.

BIBLIOGRAPHY

BOOKS

Ballentine, R. *Diet and Nutrition.* Honesdale, Pa.: Himalayan International Institute, 1978.

Berger, Stuart. *How to Be Your Own Nutritionist.* New York: Wm. Morrow, 1987.

Kirschman, J., and L. Dunne. *Nutrition Almanac.* New York: McGraw-Hill, 1984.

Long, Patricia. *The Nutritional Ages of Women.* New York: Macmillan, 1986.

Memmler, R., and D. Wood. *The Human Body in Health and Disease.* Philadelphia: J.B. Lippincott, 1983.

Pearson, Durk and Sandy Shaw. *Life Extension: A practical scientific approach.* New York: Warner Books, 1982.

Silverman, H., J. Romano, and G. Elmer. *The Vitamin Book.* New York: Bantam Books, 1985.

U.S. Surgeon General. *The Surgeon General's Report on Nutrition and Health.* Washington, D.C., 1988.

PERIODICALS

Barnett, R. A. "Nuts about selenium." *American Health,* March 1989, 149.

Beck, M. "Living with arthritis." *Newsweek,* March 20, 1989, 64–70.

Bennett, W. I. "Why diets don't work." *New Choices for the Best Years,* June 1990, 37–38.

Blackburn, G. L. "The anti-arthritis diet." *Prevention,* February 1989, 34–35.

———"Bad to the bone." *Prevention,* March 1989, 99–100.

Bloom, M. "The fats of life." *World Tennis,* September 1989, 92–95.

"Born to be fat?" *U.S. News & World Report,* May 14, 1990, 62.

Coleman, E. "The hazards of eating too little." *Women's Sports and Fitness,* March 1989, 18.

"Curtailing calories may lengthen life." *FDA Consumer,* February 1989, 3–4.

Devereaux, K. "Fiber tactics." *Women's Sports and Fitness,* March 1990, 18–19.

"Diet and your health." *Consumers' Research Magazine,* July 1989, 31–35.

"The diet-cancer link." *McCall's,* October 1989, 106.

Fackelmann, K. "Health groups find consensus on fat in diet." *Science News,* March 3, 1990, 132.

———"High carbohydrate diet may pose heart risks." *Science News,* September 16, 1989, 185.

Goode, E. E. "Getting slim." *U.S. News & World Report,* May 14, 1990, 56–58.

Grady, D. "Bad news bellies." *American Health,* May 1989, 20.

Graham, J. "Nutrition now: the hidden dangers in the foods kids eat." *Redbook,* February 1990, 114.

Green, R. "Full of beans . . . and better for it." *Health,* December 1989, 58–61.

Hackman, E. "Jump-start your day." *American Health,* April 1989, 140–142.

"High cholesterol in children." *The Saturday Evening Post,* April 1989, 42–43.

"High fiber for diabetics." *The Saturday Evening Post,* January-February 1990, 12.

Hunter, B. T. "A balancing act." *Consumers' Research Magazine,* December 1989, 8–9.

———"Appreciating individual differences." *Consumers' Research Magazine,* November 1989, 8–9.

———"Variety: for good nutrition." *Consumers' Research Magazine,* September 1989, 8–9.

Jenish, D. "A tragic obsession." *Maclean's,* October 9, 1989, 52.

"Kids' cholesterol." *Prevention,* March 1990, 20.

Kowalski, R. E. "Heart-healthy children." *Parents,* October 1989, 177.

Leblang, B. T. "A new fat." *American Health,* May 1990, 86–88.

Levin, S. "The new anticancer agenda." *Mademoiselle,* March 1989, 143–144.

McCarthy, P. "Does protein build muscles?" *American Health,* November 1989, 96.

McVeigh, G. "On the trail of nutrition's white knight." *Prevention,* February 1990, 60–64.

Meadows, S. "Improving blood glucose monitoring." *FDA Consumer,* May 1990, 32–35.

Mendoza, T. "Diet, cancer, and common sense." *Current Health,* November 1989, 18–21.

———"Mighty minerals in mini-doses." *Current Health,* December 1989, 22–25.

———"The power of iron." *Current Health,* April 1989, 14–16.

Moffat, A. S. "Fiber fracas at FASEB." *Science,* March 23, 1990, 1412.

Moller, J. "Facts about kids and cholesterol." *Good Housekeeping,* September 1989, 101.

Murray, M. "Confused about fiber?" *Reader's Digest,* July 1990, 75–78.

Nelson, C. I. "Diabetes and vitamin C." *New Choices for the Best Years,* May 1989, 15.

"Oh, those menstrual blues." *Teen,* April 1990, 20.

Palca, J. "Getting to the heart of the cholesterol debate." *Science,* March 9, 1990, 1170–1171.

Perlmutter, C. "Diet and immunity: the new frontier." *Prevention,* October 1989, 46–52.

Poppy, J. "The paunch line." *Esquire,* February 1989, 59–60.

Raeburn, P. "Beyond cholesterol." *American Health,* January-February 1990, 88.

Raloff, J. "Breast cancer rise: due to dietary fat?" *Science News,* April 21, 1990, 245.

———"Fish oil slows some developing cancers." *Science News,* June 14, 1989, 390.

———"Revised RDAs add a few good nutrients." *Science News,* October 28, 1989, 277.

"Ready, set, go! How to shape up your kids." *Ladies' Home Journal,* April 1990, 89–90.

"Reducing risk of colon cancer." *USA Today,* February 1989, 6.

Roblin, A. "New clues to the power of magnesium." *Prevention,* April 1989, 33–39.

Shockey, G. "The best quick breakfasts for active women." *Women's Sports and Fitness,* April 1989, 34–35.

———"The truth about iron." *Women's Sports and Fitness,* January-February 1989, 20-21.

Stocker-Ferguson, S. "100 top fiber foods." *Prevention,* November 1989, 73.

INDEX

EDUCATION